Herbal Indian
Perfumes and Cosmetics

Indian Medical Science Series No.-59

Herbal Indian Perfumes and Cosmetics

Vaidya Asha Ram

Sri Satguru Publications
A Division of
Indian Books Centre
Delhi, India

Published by :
Sri Satguru Publications
A Division of :
Indian Books Centre
Indological and Oriental Publishers
40/5, Shakti Nagar,
Delhi-110007
(INDIA)

All rights reserved. No part of this work covered by the Copyrights hereon may be reproduced or copied in any form or by any means— Graphics, Electronics or Mechanical including photocopying, microfiche reading without written permission from the publishers.

ISBN 81-7030-554-3

First Edition : Delhi, 1997

Published by Sunil Gupta for Sri Satguru Publications a division of Indian Books Centre, 40/5, Shakti Nagar, Delhi-110 007, India and printed at D.K.Fine Art Press, Delhi-110 052

CONTENTS

SECTION ONE : PERFUMERY INDUSTRY

1. Possibilities of the Perfumery Industry — 1
2. Classification of Perfumes — 7
3. Perfumery Materials — 11
4. Modes of Manipulation — 20
5. Principles of Manufacture — 28

SECTION TWO : ESSENTIAL EXTRACTS

6. Floral Oils — 31
7. Essential Oils — 42

SECTION THREE : ESSENCES AND OTTOS

8. Preparation of Essences — 62
9. Natural Essence — 65
10. Artificial Essences — 71
11. Preparation of Ottos — 89

SECTION FOUR : AROMATIC WATERS

12. Rose and Keora Water — 99
13. Toilet Water — 103

SECTION FIVE : HAIR OIL AND TOILET PREPARATIONS

14. Scented Hair Oils — 109
15. Taral Alta — 129
16. Toilet Preparations — 134
    Appendix — 161
    Glossary — 163

SECTION ONE
PERFUMERY INDUSTRY

CHAPTER I

POSSIBILITIES OF THE PERFUMERY INDUSTRY

From very early times mankind has been a genuine lover of perfumes of any sort which may make an agreeable appeal to his sense of smell. The pages of ancient literatures of almost all nationalities are full of references to the perfumes. Even to this day these wield a great influence over the softer emotions of the human heart and continue to play the role of a veritable source of inspiration to the poets and poetasters.

Odoriferous objects, both natural and artificial in origin, have been held in high favour all over the world, and not without foundation. There is nothing in the world which can equal them in enlivening the depressed mind and in permeating it with a new spirit of buoyancy. Many of them are, over and above, credited with actual disinfecting properties and are of immense value from the hygienic point of view. It is, therefore, no wonder that the noblemen of all countries consider the perfumes as a most necessary complement to their toileting, and even if the common people cannot afford to have them daily, they use it on every ceremonial occasion. The fair sex however has got a keen attachment for perfumes in general.

PERFUMES DEMOCRATIZED

Signs are not wanting to indicate that perfumes are coming to more general use. Formerly these were mainly reserved as luxury for the rich but now-a-days they can be indulged in by the rich and the poor alike. The reason is not far to seek. Manufacture of perfumes previously entailed most elaborate, painstaking and costly processes; consequently they were not within the reach of the common people, though they longed for these and envied their more fortunate brethren who had the means to enjoy in the luxuries of using perfumes. The complications in the manufacturing processes remain almost the same but the large scale production and organised methods of distribution and lastly, the advent of synthetic perfumes have thoroughly revolutionised the perfumery industry. Today all sorts of perfumes, ottos, essences, aromatic waters, scented hair oils, etc., can be bought cheaply; and their extended popularity must be ascribed to their cheapness and consequent accessibility to the common people who form by far the greater part of the population.

INDIAN PERFUMERY INDUSTRY

The perfumery industry is no new thing in India. Manufacture of perfumes attained a high degree of excellence in the glorious days of India. It is indeed one of the most ancient and honourable of the Indian crafts, and even now India is famous for the special types of perfumes she produces. It is no exaggeration to say that no branch of industry purely devoted to the supply of luxury is of such importance in India as that of perfumery.

That the perfumes made in India were of superb quality and caught the fancy of the then civilized world can be well gauged from the fact that the fame of her products spread out beyond the seas. In the days of Rome's magnificence Indian sandalwood, saffron and musk were regarded as essentials to the toilet of a Roman gentleman and among the chief complement of a Roman lady's *boudoir*.

FIELD FOR PERFUMERS

The field open to the perfumers is vast and varied. Indians are as fond to-day as ever of the sweet perfumes. The appearance of synthetic substitutes has doubtless affected the trade in natural perfumes, as in the dye industry, but nevertheless a very considerable demand, which instead of decreasing shows sign of increasing exists for natural perfumes even in those places which may be regarded as the chief centres of synthetic perfumery trade. The demand for scents and perfumes is increasing rapidly and there need not be any fear of lack of demand for many years to come. This demand can be met in India, if the industry is properly organised.

It is a settled fact that large quantities of wild odoriferous bodies are going to waste, and at present rose and jasmine are practically the only two plants which are being cultivated for perfumery purposes. There is, therefore, a possibility of enormously expanding this industry. But before this is done a careful and exhaustive enumeration of the odoriferous plants of the country must be compiled, as has been done in the United States. Research work conducted up to date holds out promises that when this compilation is finished, much headway now undreamt of may be made in the manufacture of perfumery, and many articles of which we are now in the complete dark and for which we have to approach the foreign countries can be manufactured in the country itself to her immense benefit and of the world as well.

VALUE OF RESEARCH WORK

It may be remarked in this connection that too much attention cannot be paid to research work. This must be carried on to ascertain the average essential oil contents of the various perfumery materials so that the nature and quality of each material may be fully known by the manufacturers. Practically nothing of the kind is done in India. It would open our eyes if we go over the minute studies made by the Western students of chemistry in the domain of perfumery. The valued results of their investigations are fully taken advantage of by the perfumers in manufacturing perfumes or attempting improvements thereon. Such study pays, and if India is to develop her indigenous perfumery industry, this side of the subject, which is now so much lost sight of and thrown off to the background, should deserve the best attention of the scientists and should be made thorough study of in the light of the Indian conditions and environments.

CULTIVATION OF PERFUMERY MATERIALS

As a counter-argument to this scheme of development of the indigenous perfumery industry, it may be advanced that the Indian spice and perfume materials are inferior to those grown elsewhere. Of course, this is a fact which must be reckoned with. But it remains to be seen how far this is due to climatic or soil conditions or to a variety of factors or what is most probable to protracted neglect in cultivation. Moreover, it is not a rare occasion where the Indian stuff has been classified as inferior to the foreign stuff on no other demerit than that the enumerator of the classifications, who is mostly a non-Indian, stamps preference on the materials of his own country to those of India. Nevertheless, this matter should meet proper attention. Stale, adulterated and improperly prepared materials have already done the industry considerable harm in foreign markets and this will take time to remedy. But if only intelligent and enterprising men with at least a working knowledge of the materials they deal in, take up the matter in earnest and work those products scientifically and if the general public be patriotic enough to support the local articles in preference to the imported ones, then there is no reason why as a group of economic products the perfumery industry should prove less valuable commercially than many other industries now regarded as more important and should not recover its proud position among the Indian exports.

SYNTHETIC VS. NATURAL PERFUMES

It is now time that India should undertake the culture of odoriferous plants, herbs, grasses and extract their essences and rare and charming perfumes from the multitudinous varieties of wild flowers which grow in profusion in our forests and valleys. It may be argued that modern synthetic perfumes have taken a good bit of profit off true or virgin flower oils; nevertheless it must also be admitted that owing to the world's demand being greater than the supply, scientists had to come to our aid with substituted stuffs, which are by no means cheap as some mistakenly believe. Besides this, perfumes made from true flower oils have a charm and fragrance of their own which is appreciated by people who are accustomed to using "perfume-par-excellence," and which fact is strongly reflected to those who do the blending of scents for powders, toilet requisites and kerchief perfumery.

It might be mentioned here that a very large proportion of crude essential oils contains oxygen and hydrocarbons, the latter as much as 90 per cent of their bulk, and these so-called "terpenes" and "sesquiterpenes," although not tasteless nor odourless contain properties which lessen their market value. With these impurities, if we may term them so, the oils are difficult to dissolve in low percentage alcohols; besides this they have a tendency to oxidise and become rancid through storage. Modern biochemistry has revealed that these unwanted properties can be successfully separated from crude essential oils without damaging their aromatic constituents which again are divided into alcohols, ethers, ketones, esters, aldehydes, etc. Oils thus treated are put on the market as terpeneless, sesquiterpeneless, supersesqui-terpeneless and carry guarantees of concentration and solubility in weak spirits, minimum cloudiness when thus mixed, and with less risks of spoilage through long storage. The time-honoured roses of Damascus and Persia, "the perfumes of Kings," is now being substituted by rose oils of Bulgaria, which is now called "the country of roses-par-excellence."

GRASS OILS

Other essential oils of commerce which have attracted moderate attention but are still neglected and being run half-heartedly are the grass oils of India which can be split up into four distinct classes and which are hopelessly confused at times. These species are Citronella, Lemon-grass, Rosha-grass and Ginger-grass, the perfumes of which are much valued by the soap and tobacco makers and their odoriferous constituents "geraniol" and "citrol" are introduced into synthetic perfumery and used for adulterating rose and reseda scents.

Although citronella can be cultured in the Central and other provinces of India, its monopoly has been handed over to Ceylon where some thousands of acres are planted out, and the island reaps rich profits annually from this oil. Rosha grass from which commercial oil known as "Palma rosa" is extracted, has stuck to the locality where it was first discovered and is fostered by the Bhils on North Khandesh (Deccan), although this grass has been found, growing wild in Berar and Nimar District in Central Provinces. Statistics prove that Rosha-grass ("Palma rosa") oil exported from the port of Bombay has attracted buyers from England, France, America, Germany, Holland and Switzerland.

A wider field is thus open to investors of similar undertakings. Oils of lemon grass are chiefly distilled in Travancore, on the cottage industry scale with crude stills, and a valuable essential oil of leaf geranium (known as Bourbon "Rose-Geranium oil") has been cultured and distilled at Yercaud, in the Sheveroy Hills of Southern India.

MEDICINAL OILS

Similarly valuable medicinal oils and perfumery extracts could be had from other plants and spices of India, for instance the Citrus tree gives three valuable oils, i.e., "Bergamot" from the rinds of the fruit, "Petitgrain" from the leaves and "Neroli" (or orange blossom) from the flowers. Oils from kernels of almonds, apricots, peaches give almond oils and "Benzaldehyde," and other seeds such as anethi, ajwan, aniseed, clove, cardamom, etc., give us valuable essential oils which are retailed at fairly high prices because they are clarified and re-imported into the country by foreigners.

CHAPTER II

CLASSIFICATION OF PERFUMES

Quite an innumerable variety of scents and perfumes is manufactured for the Indian market. The varied combinations of the hundreds of essential principles of perfumes give rise to numerous preparations which though not materially differing in kind are each characterised by a distinct odour. Almost every day a new kind of scented preparation is launched upon the market. Some of them charmingly appeal to the taste of the people and have thus a more or less prosperous career assured, while the others fail to catch the popular fancy and are consequently given up in time.

CHARACTERISTICS OF PERFUMES

But unlike the varieties, the principal classes into which all articles of perfumery can be grouped and the chief purposes they are meant to serve are rather limited in number. But whatever be the purpose which the perfumes are intended for, they must as a general criterion emit an agreeable odour so that the user may derive a unique gratification of the senses from their employment. All classes of perfumery irrespective of their special properties and even medicinal effects, must be characterised by this general criterion, and one of the objects of the manufacturer should be to arrive at a preparation which, besides possessing special properties appertaining to the class, which it belongs to, combines a delightful and refreshing odour by proper selection of the raw materials and judicious manipulation.

OTTO—THE QUEEN OF PERFUMES

The principal class into which the perfumes may be grouped is the otto, or the concentrated principle of the natural flowers. Nothing can stand in comparison with the sublime fragrance the ottos yield and if their popularity has declined of late it is not for any inherent defect in their composition, but for the high costs of the preparations. Their use among the noblemen remains undiminished and in fact these are employed in small doses in the preparation of chief commercial essences which flood the market now-a-days. From the Indian point of view the otto is the queen of the perfumery preparation and its manufacture has engaged the best attention from the Indians for many centuries. The industry is now situated in the northern part of India, specially in Jaunpur, Ghazipur and Quetta.

The manufacture of the ottos has in view the extraction of the essential principle of the natural flowers, which yield a fragrance of the highest degree of excellence, surpassed by none else in the world. The flowers wither away in course of time and with them their fragrance also dies. It is the perfumer's art to extract the fragrance apart from the flowers for applications in the various arts and industries and preserve it for future use.

FLORAL OILS

The next in importance from the Indian point of view is the floral oil. These are delicious preparations of oils laden with the scents of fresh-blown flowers. These possess unique hair dressing qualities, inimitable fragrance, cooling and soothing effects and are strictly non-injurious to health or the growth of hair. For these reasons floral oils are in extensive demand all over the country for toilet purposes by the men of fashion.

The floral oil industry has of course met a setback on the advent of the so-called scented hair oils which are simply vegetable or mineral oils surcharged with synthetic essential oils and are by no means non-injurious. The industry can nevertheless hold its own against the commercial scented hair oils. Virtually pure floral oils are widely employed as basis in the manufacture of the finely scented hair oils.

AROMATIC WATERS

Aromatic waters should occupy the next place in order of importance. They embrace quite a number of products possessing medicinal properties or sometimes simple aroma. The principal of these is the rose water which requires no introduction to the public. Its wide applications in the arts, industries, medicine, and even in confectionery making are too well-known to require any recapitulation. Then there is the *keora* water, a watery preparation laden with the distinctive smell of the *keora* flowers. There is a pretty big demand for this article, though compared with that for rose water this pales into insignificance. This is used for scenting the drinking water and adding a peculiar flavour to the *sherbat* preparations. These two are of purely indigenous origin and are both largely employed for toilet purposes. But in foreign countries much interest attaches to the manufacture of Eau de Cologne and lavender water, and in fact in those countries the perfumers are really tested by the standard of these waters they are capable of producing. In this country also they are partly used for the preparation of toilet articles and are prescribed by the doctors for cooling effect in cases of high fever.

ESSENTIAL OILS

The preparation of essential oils is another important branch of perfumery, and this should warrant greater attention than hitherto paid to it. India abounds in odoriferous substances which may be made to yield valuable essential oils with their characteristic odours and properties. Some of them are moreover found to possess valuable medicinal properties. This industry is now neglected in India. Yet quite a big quantity of essential oils is annually imported into India from foreign countries while the Indian raw materials are allowed to run to waste. They have their wide applications in perfumery, medicine and art and if the indigenous perfumery industry is to be placed on an organised footing, attention should be concentrated on this subject.

ESSENCE—THE COMMONER'S PERFUME

The classes of perfumes mentioned above are all indigenous to India. But there is still another kind of perfume which commonly goes by the name of essences. Like ottos they are used for their sweet smell by all lovers of perfumes. Essences are used as handkerchief perfumes and as scents for dresses. The demand for the excellent preparations is as big as ever.

Essences from artificial sources for handkerchief scents are now-a-days in fashion on account of their harmonious scent and cheapness. Perfumers have to bring out their ripe experience to get a preparation which will appeal to the popular fancy and will at the same time be as pleasing and durable as possible. Their preparation thus will tax the best brain of the perfumers.

MISCELLANEOUS CLASSES

Besides these, there are other classes of perfumes of minor importance, such as pomades, face powders, scented hair oils, dry perfumes, satchet powders, hair lotions, etc., etc. Snow creams, face powders, etc., also play an important part in making up the toileting of the fair sex. The demand for these articles in the Indian market is ever on the increase. If really good preparations can be made and offered in the market in an attractive style, there is no reason why the Indian perfumers will not be benefited by commanding a significant part of the perfumery trade.

Another toilet product is the taral alta, a brilliant red liquid colour for painting the feet of the ladies. Its preparation is easy and profitable too.

CHAPTER III

PERFUMERY MATERIALS

To be a successful manufacturer, every perfumer should be fully familiar with the nature and properties of the hundreds of raw materials he makes use of in the manufacture of his products. Simple knowledge helping the identification of the raw materials should not be by any means considered sufficient. It is incumbent on the perfumer to possess a thorough scientific knowledge of these articles, their chemical properties and their behaviour to one another. It is a common observation that scents are considerably modified, rounded off and even spoilt when they come into combination with some special types of scented materials. The more is one's acquaintance with these facts, the greater is his chance of getting the most excellent preparations. When the perfumer is so equipped he will be in a position to guess what perfumes should be combined together and in what quantities so that when the blending is completed the preparation yields a fragrance, harmonious and free from discords. For a novice in the line it is simply impossible to say what substances are sympathetic or antipathetic towards one another, and it is only experience that matters in such circumstances.

SENSE OF SMELL IN PERFUMERS

Over and above this, the perfumer should have an extremely sensitive sense of smell. The characteristic odours given out by each of these raw materials should be individually studied and known. He should be qualified to discriminate the several ingredients from any given perfumed preparation and detect if the blending is all that could be desired or can be improved upon. He should also be able to find out the jarring elements in the composition.

Broadly speaking, the aromatic substances can be classified under three groups:

CLASSES OF RAW PERFUMES

1. Materials of purely vegetable origin.

2. Materials of purely animal origin.
3. Synthetic or artificial perfumes.

SOURCES OF VEGETABLE PERFUMES

The most common example of an aromatic substance of vegetable origin is the flower which is unsurpassed in the freshness of the perfume which is said by the scientists to be due to the minute traces of essential oils present in its petals. Besides flowers, perfumes are capable of extraction from various herbs, roots, barks, leaves, stems, fruits and other parts of vegetable plants. For instance, perfumes can be obtained from the flowers of cloves, etc; leaves and stems of patchouli, cinnamon, etc. barks of cassia, cinnamon etc.; woods of cedar, sandal, etc.; roots of sassafras, vetiver etc.; rhizomes of ginger, orris, etc.; fruits of lemon, etc.; seeds of bitter almonds, anise, etc.; gums or resinous exudations from myrrh, olibanum, etc., etc. Various spices also furnish a rich variety of perfume materials.

It is thus apparent that the fragrance is not confined to full-blown flowers only but may be suitably derived from all organs of the plants. Mention may also be made here that some plants also are capable of yielding more than one odour quite distinct and characteristic in nature. The most commonly noted example is no doubt the orange tree from which three distinct perfumes may be secured, one from the leaves, one from the fruits and one from the rind of the fruit.

ANIMAL PERFUMES

Perfumes are also obtained from animal origin. These occur almost exclusively as glandular secretions and enter into commerce in their natural state. The chief among them are musk, ambergris, castor and civet.

Animal perfumes are specially distinguished for their property of giving permanence to the odour of other bodies with which these are mixed. The odour they possess is also characterised by wide diffusion hardly surpassed by anything else. They are held in very high esteem and are, therefore, liable to indiscriminate adulteration. Various attempts have been made to reproduce their peculiar odours synthetically or by the combination of scents but so far all trials have been fruitless and adulteration continues rife as before. But it must be remembered that in perfumery making, adulterated animal perfumes are of rarely any importance; they do neither improve the tone of the preparation nor render the odour persistent.

Musk

Musk, to cite an example, is obtained from musk deer and possesses an inimitable odour. Its presence even in small doses is capable of detection by perfumers. But this being a rare object and valuable, it undergoes considerable adulteration with dried blood, animal excrement, earth, etc. The extent of these additions varies from 25 per cent to 75 per cent of the gross weight of the mixture. The blood is dried by the heat of steam or on water bath, then reduced to coarse powder, and triturated with the genuine musk in a mortar along with a few drops of liquid ammonia. It is then either replaced in the empty pots, or it is put into bottles and sold as grain musk. There are only three certain ways of detecting this fraud, viz., by the inferiority of the odour, by an assay for the iron contained in the blood, or by the microscope. Genuine musk often becomes nearly inodorous by keeping, but recovers its smell on being exposed to the vapour of ammonia, or by being moistened with ammonia water. The following tests may also be applied.

Pure musk, by trituration or digestion with boiling water, loses about 75 per cent of its weight, and the boiling solution, after precipitation with nitric acid, is nearly colourless. A solution of acetate of lead, and a cold decoction of galls, also precipitate the solution; but one of corrosive sublimate does not disturb it. The ashes left after the incineration of pure musk are neither red nor yellow, but grey, and should not exceed 5 per cent to 6 per cent. One of the best solvents for musk is ether. Musk has also been prepared in the laboratory synthetically but its odour has not yet been exactly copied so far.

Ambergris

Ambergris is found in the intestines of spermaceti whales and is much prized in perfumery. Its presence even in minute traces is perceptible and permeates the whole with an exalting odour. Its tincture is hence sometimes made the basis in the preparation of ottos, essences, etc.

Ambergris is solid, opaque, ash-coloured, streaked or variegated, fatty, inflammable, remarkably light and highly odorous. It has a pleasant musk-like odour, which is supposed to be derived from the squid (Sepia moschata) on which the animal feeds, the horny beaks of which are often found embedded in the masses. The odour is peculiar and not easily described or imitated, of a very diffusive and penetrating character, and perceptible in minute quantities. Ambergris is rugged on the surface; does not effervesce with acids; melts at 140°-150°F into a yellowish resin-like mass; at 212°F sublimes as a white vapour; very soluble in alcohol, ether, and the volatile and fixed oils. It appears to be a body analogous to cholesterine. Its specific gravity is 0.780 to 0.926.

Due to the high price of genuine ambergris it is very frequently, if not nearly always, adulterated. When quite pure and of the best quality: 1. It is nearly wholly soluble in hot alcohol and ether, and yields about 85 per cent of ambreine; 2. It almost wholly volatilises at a moderate heat, and when burnt leaves no notable quantity of ashes; a little of it exposed in a silver spoon melts without bubble or scum; and on the heated point of a knife it is rapidly and entirely dissipated; 3. It is easily punctured with a heated needle, and on withdrawing it, not only should the odour be immediately evolved, but the needle should come out clean, without anything adhering to it; 4. Acids, except nitric acid, act feebly on it; alkalies combine with it and form a soap. The Chinese are said to try its genuineness by scraping it fine upon the top of boiling tea. It should dissolve and diffuse itself generally. Black or white ambergris is bad while the smooth and uniform one is generally fictitious.

Civet

Civet is another animal perfume having very strong smell and hence should only be used in a diluted state in manufacturing perfumery. If added in excess, the smell is unbearable and even nauseous. But when added in measured doses, it imparts a most pleasant fragrance to the preparation and makes it lasting.

Castor

Castor, an unctuous substance derived from the beaver, is also incorporated in small quantities only in making perfumery.

It gives a black tincture, which added in big quantities would discolour the whole preparation. Its odour specially improves on keeping.

SYNTHETIC PERFUMES

The third form of perfumes is, however, the synthetic perfume, which constitutes a veritable romance of organic chemical research. Its evolution has brought about a complete revolution in the perfumery industry. The perfumes are not directly manufactured from the odoriferous bodies but are derived by a chain of chemical processes perfected in the laboratories. For example, vanillin is derived from benzene, salicylates from salicylic acid which in its turn is made from phenol; benzyl esters, phenylethyl alcohols, benzoic esters are derived from toluene; xylene musk and ketone musk are both derivatives of metaxylene; methyl ether, ethyl ether, indol, etc., are obtained from treatment of naphthalene; coumarin, musk ambrette, anisic esters are derived from cresol; etc., etc.

A number of synthetic perfumes are derived from vegetable essential oils; for example, terpineol from turpentine; citral, ionone from lemon grass oil; geraniol from Java citronella oil; rhodinol from geranium oil; geraniol from palmarosa oil; safrol, iso-safrol, henotropine from camphor oil; anethol from aniseed oil; eugenol from clove oil; linalol from rosewood oil; cinnamic alcohol from styrax; etc., etc.

The characteristic odours derived from these synthetic perfumes are given below:

Amyl acetate gives the odour of pear, apple and banana; bornyl acetate, jasmine; linalyl acetate, bergamot; benzyl alcohol, slight jasmine; phenyl ethyl alcohol, rose; benzoic aldehyde, bitter almonds; cinnamic aldehyde, cassia and cinnamon; citral, lemongrass; citronellal, citronella grass; citronellol, rose; ethyl anthranillate, neroli; eugenol, cloves; florentinol, orris; geraniol; rose; geranyl formate, rose geranium; heliotropin, heliotrope; ionone violet; geranyl acetate, wildrose; jasmindol, jasmine; lavandol, lavender; methyl salicylate, wintergreen; muguet, lily of the valley; terpeniol, lilac, lily; tonquinol, tonquin bean, musk; vanillin, vanilla; yara yara, neroli; zibethin, civet.

The range of synthetic products at the disposal of the perfumer at the present time is extensively wide and many of the peculiar aromas characterising certain natural bodies have been, exactly or with a close approximation, reproduced in the laboratory. The underlying principle of manufacturing synthetic perfumes has also been utilised by the perfumers and those of roses, violet, etc., have not yet been derived with any close fidelity.

Now-a-days essential oils and synthetic derivatives representing the oils are freely used as substitutes for one another. As for instance, oil of orange is a natural product while oil of neroli is prepared synthetically but they are so very identical in their constituents that they are freely interchangeable. Vanillin from pods of vanilla and artificial vanillin from eugenol are also similarly interchangeable; oil of bitter almonds with benzaldehyde; and so on.

The synthetic products are not used alone but are suitably blended and modified by the perfumers before they reach the real consumers. They are mixed together in suitable proportions to imitate the natural perfumes of certain flowers. For example, the fragrance of the rose is not produced by a single synthetic perfume but phenylethyl alcohol mixed with geraniol, citronellol, essences extracted from various plants, and several other synthetic products yields an oil, which is a very passable imitation of otto of rose.

MODIFIERS AND FIXERS

The raw materials for the perfumery industry may be classified from another standpoint under three groups: the distinctive odours, the modifiers and the fixers. The distinctive odours most relished are those of rosemary, patchouli, bergamot, ylang musk, lily of the valley, heliotrope, narcissus, geranium, hyacinth, benzoin, etc., etc. But sometimes these fail to appeal properly to the sense of smell. They are, in such case, combined with modifiers which mellow, soften down or temper, as it is called, the smell of the distinctive odour. Thirdly, the essential oils used in combination to secure the harmonious blend of any perfumery preparation possess unequal rates of evaporation, i.e., some of them are more volatile than the rest. Hence the need of adding some agents which would prevent the unequal evaporation of the individual perfumes, render the odour persistent by reducing the rate of evaporation and at the same time maintain the predominant note of their fragrance. These agents are known as fixers or fixative agents or binders.

The group of bodies from which suitable fixatives for any perfume can be selected is a large one. Various perfume materials known as tincture or extracts are added as fixatives, some of which are pleasantly aromatic, some disagreeable and some others neutral. The principal of these are benzoin, peru balsam, tolu balsam, storax, myrrh, patchouli, khus, sandalwood, musk, ambergris, benzyl, benzoate, ethyl phthalate and glyceryl acetate.

ALCOHOL

Another commodity which largely enters into the composition of essences, ottos, essential oils, aromatic waters, etc., is alcohol which is variously known as spirits, rectified spirit, absolute alcohol, spirit of wine, according to the purity of the stuff. The ardent spirits which are obtained by distilling fermented liquors consist mainly of three ingredients, alcohol, water and a little oil or resin, to which they owe their flavour and colour. When these liquids are redistilled the first portion that comes over is a fine, light, transparent fluid, known in commerce by the name of rectified spirits. Specific gravity of highly rectified spirit is not less than 0.8200 and is generally more. Alcohol cannot, by this process, be deprived of the whole of the water with which it is combined; but by redistillation with not hydrochlorate of lime, it is procured of the specific gravity of 0.739 at 60°F. In this state it is the strongest that can be procured, and it is, therefore, called pure or absolute alcohol. The alcohol of commerce, or spirit of wine is never so strong as this; its specific gravity is seldom under 0.8370. In this state it is fragrant, limpid, colourless, volatile, inflammable, and of a pungent, agreeable taste. It combines with water in every degree; and the proportion of it present in common spirits can be best judged by their specific gravity. The specific gravity of pure alcohol being 0.7939 at 60°F and that of water 1.000, it follows, that the lighter a spirit is, the stronger it is. Proof spirit is a mixture of equal bulks of alcohol and water. When spirits are weaker than this they are said to be underproof; when stronger, to be aboveproof; thus, "10 underproof" signifies that every 100 gallons of that spirit would require to have 10 gallons of water abstracted from it to bring it up to proof; and "10 overproof" means that every 100 gallons contains too little water by 10 gallons.

To get brilliant results the manufacturers should make it a point to use rather old alcohol which has been left sufficiently long to mature.

In order to reduce the price of the preparations requiring the use of alcohol, manufacturers use spirit chloroform in place of alcohol.

AUXILIARY MATERIALS

Besides these odorous raw materials, the perfumer makes use of a number of auxiliary substances such as water, alcohol, fixed oils for making hair oils, fats for pomades, etc. To be successful, the manufacturer should devote particular attention to their purity and must also be conversant with their properties and purposes they are intended for.

Fixed oils employed in making floral oils and essential preparations should be in a refined condition. They should be of a thin consistency as far as possible and if required they may be refined, filtered and finally deodorised. (See Page 21).

The most used of the fixed oils are the sesamum oil and olive oil but for making scented hair oils other oils like almond oil, coconut oil, white oil, etc., are made use of. The same remarks should apply in the case of these oils as well.

Glycerine and fats are also used in making perfumed cosmetics, creams, etc. These should also be of pure form and high quality.

Diverse spices and raw materials also enter into the composition of the essential oils. These require to be selected with utmost care. These are to be bruised, mashed or powdered according to the requirements they are called upon to fulfil. Fineness of a powder is technically determined by its free passage through meshed sieves.

	Diameter of particles passing through a
No. 40	mesh sieve is less than 0.38 millimeters.
" 50	" " " 0.28 "
" 60	" " " 0.23 "
" 80	" " " 0.17 "
" 100	" " " 0.14 "
" 120	" " " 0.12 "
" 150	" " " 0.09 "
" 200	" " " 0.07 "

CHAPTER IV

MODES OF MANIPULATION

Perfect manipulations are essential to the success of the perfumers. Most of the raw materials requires treatment before being employed in the making of the perfumes. Water to be used in the making of perfumes should be distilled. Alcohol is to be deodorised. The flowers are to be cleaned from dirt, dust, etc.; the stalks and green parts are to be removed; the rotten parts are to be rejected. The roots, stems and other hard odoriferous substances are to be cut into small bits, bruised, sunned or dried. Dried bodies are to be moistened to cause them to open or unroll. Sesame, castor and other oils as obtained from the market are not in a sufficiently pure state to be used as raw materials in perfumery and are liable to get sticky on keeping. They are far from being sufficiently bleached and deodorised for ordinary use. These are to be refined before use.

WATER

For best results water to be used in making perfumery must be specially treated. Ordinary water cannot be used as it is not sufficiently clean and contains a number of germs which would go to vitiate the preparation in the end. Unclean water causes turbidity which should by all means be guarded against. Water, therefore, before being used, must be filtered and freed from all suspended impurities and contaminations. Distilled water is, however, the most suited and should be employed whenever possible. Special stress should be laid by the manufacturers on the use of soft water, i.e., water which forms lather with soap at once.

DEODORISATION OF ALCOHOL

Alcohol largely enters into the preparation of essences and ottos. This also requires careful attention. Crude alcohol as found in commerce contains a lot of foreign matters with characteristic odours which it is difficult to mask. Only rectified spirit is, therefore, recommended, specially when a high quality is desired.

On many occasions, however the perfumers specially treat the alcohol to render it deodorised so that the risk of spoiling the perfumes in the dissolved extracts may be minimised. Usually one gram of benzoin R added to one litre of alcohol serves to neutralise the characteristic odour of alcohol in a few weeks. To ensure perfect deodorisation, 1 gram each of benzoin and tolu and 1/2 gram of olibanum are added to a litre of alcohol and the whole is allowed to stand for a month. Such treatment is especially needed when the specified alcoholic scent does not agree with the perfumes added and in the preparation of Eau de Cologne.

Another method of deodorising alcohol consists in adding half an ounce of powdered quicklime, 2 oz. of powdered alum and 1 oz. of wood charcoal to one gallon of alcohol. The whole is allowed to stand for a few days and then filtered.

Another method of maturing ordinary alcohol follows:

Alcohol	1 gall.
Powdered slaked lime	4 dr.
Powdered alum	2 dr.
Spirit of nitrous ether	1 dr.

Mix the lime and alum and add them to the alcohol shaking the mixture well together, then add the spirit of nitrous ether and set aside for some days, shaking occasionally; finally filter.

REFINING OF OILS

The impurities in freshly expressed oils are partly in suspension and partly in solution. These consist chiefly of dirt, fragments of vegetable fibre, and mucilaginous and albuminous substances. A portion of them rapidly deposits when the oil is allowed to stand, and the upper liquid may then be drawn off from the sediment and subjected to filtration or to further refining processes.

REMOVAL OF SUSPENDED MATTER

In some cases a simple filtration, after standing for a short time, is sufficient to render the oil brilliant. The oil is made to pass through a piece of properly folded blotting or filter paper fitted on a funnel or through a piece of flannel, made two or three fold. The operation may be repeated for better results. But when there is an excess of albuminous matter, the oils are not sufficiently clear after passing through the filter. In such cases various methods are employed to coagulate or precipitate the matters before filtration, such as dry heat, introduction of fine jets of steam, or the addition of a small quantity of insoluble powder (e.g., fuller's earth or kieselguhr) which as it subsides attracts and carries down simultaneously the particles of the gum-like mucilage.

REMOVAL OF MUCILAGINOUS MATTERS

On a small scale the removal of mucilage is effected by heating the oil in a special type of cast iron pan built into a flue in such a way that the hot gases strike the sides rather than the bottom of the pan. The vegetable matter on precipitation sinks to the bottom, and if the heat is applied just at the bottom of the boiling pan, the vegetable matter becomes charred and thus injuriously affects the quality and colour of the oil. Heating must be done very carefully to drive off all the moisture present in the oil. In no case overheating should be done. If the temperature becomes comparatively high, a little water should be added to the oil. When free from moisture the oil is allowed to cool and settle.

On a comparatively large scale, the operation can be carried out in steam-jacketed tanks having a jacket all round the sides, but not on the bottom. The bottom should be conical in shape. The vessel is also provided with a mechanical agitator. Heating is generally done by passing steam at atmospheric pressure through the jacket. When free from moisture the oil is allowed to cool so that the solid impurities are collected in the groove of the conical portion.

On a small scale the operation is carried out on water bath with fairly good results.

The Filter Press

A convenient form of mechanical refining is afforded by a filter press. A common form of filter press consists of a hydraulic press containing a series of communicating plates with rims raised so as to form a space into which filter cloths may be fitted.

After adjusting the filter press the oil is pumped into the press at the right-hand end, and is made to flow through chambers between the plates and is collected in a trough. After using the press for a good length of time the filter cloths are found to be clogged with various impurities so that it is desirable to remove press filter cloths occasionally. The filter cloths after removal from the press are transferred to a washing machine, where they are treated with a hot dilute solution of caustic soda which combining with the oil, produces soap and so cleanses the cloths from mucilage and dirt.

The materials used as filtering media include sand, kieselguhr, Spanish clay, fuller's earth, animal charcoal, paper pulp, and a mixture of wood and vegetable fibres disintegrated into a pulp.

REMOVAL OF FATTY ACIDS

To remove the fatty acids, the oil is treated with a sufficient quantity of caustic soda solution of known strength and at the same time the temperature of the oil is carefully regulated. It must be understood that more caustic soda has to be added to the oil than is theoretically necessary to neutralise the percentage of free acid revealed by actual analysis. The surplus soda does not, however, attack the neutral oil unless the amount is allowed to stand for some hours to permit the soap, soda solution and any remaining mucilage to sink to the bottom, while the oil occupies the upper layers as a clear liquid, which is then drawn off for further treatment. The solid residue left in the kettle should not be thrown away but be sold to the soap maker as "soap stock."

To facilitate the setting out of the soap, etc., from the oil, common salt is sometimes thrown into the oil kettle. Soda soap being insoluble in salt water separates out. The clear oil thus obtained is next washed with water to remove all traces of soda from it. Thereafter it is treated in a vacuum still to drive off any volatile fatty acids, still adhering to it as well as the last traces of moisture, which finds its way at the time of washing.

Mention should, however, be made that great care need be exercised in using caustic soda for the above purpose. Being possessed of high caustic properties, it is liable to attack the good oil, converting it into soap. In that case only a small percentage of the pure oil can be recovered.

Washing soda, wood ash and potash carbonate may also be used to remove the rancidity. As a working rule it may be stated that to neutralise 1 per cent of acidity present in 1,000 lbs. of oil, 1.9 lbs. of washing soda or 1.4 lbs. of caustic soda, 65 lbs. of wood ash and 2.5 lbs. of potash carbonate will be required.

REMOVAL OF DISSOLVED IMPURITIES

In the removal of dissolved impurities alkali solutions, milk of lime, or magnesia are reagents in common use, while dilute sulphuric acid is sometimes employed to clarify linseed and certain fish oils for industrial purposes.

BLEACHING AND DEODORISING OILS

The purification of oil may be effected by washing the oil with water to which aluminium sulphate has been added in the proportion of about 3/4 oz. to 220 gallons per degree of hardness. This forms with the lime in the water a bulky colloidal precipitate which serves to bleach and clarify the oil.

Treatment of oil with fuller's earth, animal charcoal, etc., not only helps to bleach the oil but also assists in deodorising it to a certain extent. The oil to be bleached is poured into a steam-jacketed mixing still provided with a mechanical agitator and a steam coil. Before pouring the oil, the vessel is heated by admitting steam to the jacket, care being taken to see that the steam condensed may drain out of the jacket. The oil already heated to a temperature of 150°F is run into the kettle until this is filled to within 4 inches of the top cover; the mixing gear being put to work in the meantime in order to agitate the oil and drive off any moisture contained therein. The successful working of the process depends to a considerable extent upon the complete absence of moisture, and it is essential, therefore, that the oil, fuller's earth, filter cloths, and the whole of the apparatus should be as dry as possible. The fuller's earth in fine powder is added as soon as the oil in the kettle is at a temperature of 150°F. The quantity of earth necessary usually varies between 2½ and 5 per cent, but it may be more or less according to the quality of the oil being treated. The exact proportion can be determined by an experiment on a small scale. This experimental test will also enable the most suitable temperature to be ascertained. The process should be worked at the minimum temperature found to give the desired result, as there is less danger of an earthy flavour being imparted to the oil at a lower temperature. After a few minutes' agitation the earth will be uniformly and intimately mixed with the oil, and the few pumps on the filter press should be started to work so that the whole batch is pumped into the filter press in the shortest possible time. As soon as the filtering operation is finished, the fuller's earth remaining in the press should be steamed out in order to recover as much as possible of the oil contained in the earth.

Immediately after steaming out the press must be opened and the plates separated from each other, so as to leave an equal space between all the plates. The heat contained in the iron plates will dry the cloths so that the fuller's earth already deposited on them should be removed. The oil present in the fuller's earth can then be separated easily.

When dealing with viscous oils, such as castor, linseed, etc., the filter press should be previously heated to ensure that the temperature of the oil while passing through the filter press is not reduced below the point necessary for efficient filtration.

Many other methods of bleaching oils by means of chemicals or otherwise are practised. It is not necessary for us to discuss these in detail in the treatise. We need only remark that one of the oldest and very satisfactory methods is to expose the oil to the action of animal charcoal, sunlight and air. This process results in the natural oxidation of the colouring matter, and is extensively adopted in the case of linseed, and poppy seed oils. It is, of course, a very slow method.

The principle consists in treating the oil with animal charcoal, preferably in a powdered condition. Not more than 1 seer of charcoal should be added to 10 seers of the oil. After this the mouth of the vessel containing the oil and charcoal is covered to prevent dirt, dust, etc., from coming in. The whole is then exposed to sunlight for a fortnight at least. The oil is then filtered through flannel when perfectly clean and limpid oil will be obtained.

FILTRATION

In making perfumery articles the manufacturer is often called upon to filter his products. For the purpose, filter papers are cut into circles and folded to make a conical cup to fit into the funnel, the inside of which may be ridged and grooved so that the filtered liquid can easily drain away. The liquid to be filtered should not be poured right into the middle of the funnel. The filter paper should be first moistened by dropping a few drops of the liquid on all sides of the paper and then the liquid can be poured along one side of the funnel. A receiver should be put under the orifice of the funnel to receive the dripping liquid. For liquids very difficult to filter a flannel strainer exactly fitting the funnel is often used.

UTILISING WASTE FILTER PAPER

Mention may be made here that special thin paper is required for filtering resinous liquids such as solution of gum resins in perfumery. The addition of carbonate of magnesia (filtering powder), talc, kaolin, however, assists the process.

The waste filter papers are not thrown away. The precipitate may be scraped and made into satchet powders. Sometimes the used filter papers are stored in a closed vessel containing 95 per cent alcohol which is stirred occasionally when cheap perfumes are obtained. Filter papers are also sometimes simply pressed and utilised in solid form as best as they can be.

COLORATION

The coloration of the perfumed articles is a problem to the manufacturers. Usually floral oils, ottos and essences go uncoloured. Hair oils however are always coloured. Alkanet root is the chief natural colour used but nowadays aniline colours (oil soluble) are in use. Taral alta is made with brilliant scarlet dye, e.g., rhodamine, eosine, etc.

The typical dyes used in toilet preparations follow:

Blue—Alizarine Delphenol, Chlorazol Blues, Coomassie, Disulphine Blue, Induline, Paramine Sky Blue, etc.

Brown—Bismarck Brown, Chlorazol, Dark Brown Basic, Paramine Brown, Phenylene Brown, Oil Brown.

Green—Alizarine Cyanine Green, Basic Green, Chlorazol Greens, Naphthol Green, Methylene Green, Oil Green, Paramine Green.

Orange—Acid Phosphine R, Acridine Orange, Chlorazol, Chrysoidine N.S., Paramine Fast Orange.

Red—Acid Magenta N., Acid Scarlet, Aurine, Azo acid, Benzo-purpurine, Carmoisine, Congo Rubine, Crocine Scarlet, Sapranine, Rosophenine, Ponceau, Heliotrope 2 R.

Violet—Coomassie Violet, Methyl Violets, Chlorazol Violet, Oil Violet, Paramine Fast Violet.

Yellow—Acid Yellow, Acridine Yellow, Auramine Yellow, Naphthol Yellow, Paramine Fast Yellow, Paraphenine G, Primuline, Tartrazine.

WATER BATH AND STEAM BATH

Instead of applying direct heat to the perfume-bearing substances, which might get injured, these are often subjected to water bath and steam bath. The distinction between water bath and steam bath should be distinctly understood. In the former case the vessel in which the extract is under preparation is suspended in hot water contained in a bigger vessel heated from below. In the latter case the vessel in which the extract is being made is put at the top of the other vessel containing water and heated from below for generating steam. The upper vessel fits into the mouth of the lower vessel and is heated by steam and not by boiling water as in the former case.

CHAPTER V

PRINCIPLES OF MANUFACTURE

The principle of making extracts from perfume-bearing substances differs widely according to their nature. But essentially these may be classed under the following categories:

1. Expression.
2. Maceration.
3. Digestion.
4. Infusion.
5. Absorption or Enfleurage.
6. Distillation.
7. Extraction from volatile solvents.

PRESSING

Extraction of perfumes from the aromatic bodies is generally made through the agency of non-volatile or volatile solvents with or without the agency of heat, but sometimes the extract is obtained by simple expression. The raw materials are packed in a strong cloth bag and the oils are expressed in a press by strong pressure. The bodies are sometimes squeezed with great force in a small squeezer and the extract is collected from below. When manufacturing on a large scale squeezing presses may be used for the purpose. The oils contain water and foreign matters which may be easily separated by settling in a separating funnel. The separated oil may be further clarified by filtering through cloth or filter paper. Generally, aromatic bodies which are fresh, rich in oils, plump and soft with juicy cells inside such as, citrus, lemon, peel of oranges etc., are most suited for such treatment.

MACERATION

Maceration consists in extracting the odoriferous principle by steeping the substance in some suitable solvent. The process is adopted in extracting perfumes in case when the natural perfume is volatile and is not capable of bearing high temperature. The substance is, therefore, steeped in some fixed oil or spirit and sometimes in water and left undisturbed in the temperature of the room or kept at 65°C upon a steam bath for 48 hours. Be it said that for the success of this operation the perfumes should be readily soluble. The duration of the process should depend upon the nature of the substance and the solubility of its constituents. Sometimes maceration is also adopted as an initial step for further treatment.

DIGESTION

Digestion consists in extracting the fragrant element by the aid of warm liquids, which are not allowed to attain boiling temperatures. One usually submits to digestion only those substances which are very slow to yield up their perfume and for which employment of heat to some extent is indispensable. If a manufacturer is, however, pressed for time and wishes to shorten the process, he may raise the temperature and stir the mixture constantly.

INFUSION

Non-volatile bodies may be subjected for extraction of their perfumes to the process of infusion which consists in steeping the substances in some boiling liquid in a closed vessel to prevent evaporation of the perfumed substances if any. The period of infusion varies according to the greater or less solubility in the solvent of the body to be extracted.

ABSORPTION OR ENFLEURAGE PROCESS

The method of extraction by enfleurage is widely in vogue in India. The inherent principle of working is as follows: A layer of the flowers from which the perfume is to be derived is placed on a clear masonry floor, to a thickness of half an inch; over this is spread a layer of *til* seed, a quarter of an inch thick, then another layer of flowers and another of seed, and so on till eight or ten altogether have been laid down. This heap is left all night; next morning the flowers are removed, and the seeds are left all day in the sunshine. In the evening the process is repeated, layers of fresh flowers are laid down alternating with layers of the now-partly-perfumed seeds, and this goes on for ten days. The scented *til* is then put in bags or jars till sufficient seed has been collected for pressing. The seed can be kept thus stored for a long time without losing the scent. As a rule, it is laid by for about a year, since the pressing can be done at any time under cover, while the perfuming can be carried on only during the dry season in the open air. The scented seeds are finally ground in a *ghani* or indigenous oil press.

DISTILLATION

The method of distillation is widely in use in preparing perfumes and specially geranium, lavender, neroli, rose, citronella, grass, lemon grass, eucalyptus, cloves, cinnamon, cardamom, sandalwood. In fact the process may be employed when the raw materials are not rich in oils and cannot be extracted by pressure. The process chiefly consists in heating the substance in some liquid in a closed vessel, called a distillation still, provided with an elongated opening on the side for the escape of the volatile perfume. This long tube helps the condensation of the steam charged with the perfume. The perfume is collected and concentrated. The condensed liquid is allowed to fall into a glass Florentine flask when the excess of perfumed water passes out into bottles through one tube and the essential oil through another tube. The oil is further clarified by filtering.

EXTRACTION BY VOLATILE SOLVENTS

Carefully refined petroleum ether, vaporizing completely at 50 deg. C. and possessing no unpleasant smell is the best solvent. The raw materials are treated with the petroleum ether which is then drawn into the still, evaporated, condensed and allowed to collect in the vessel containing the raw materials leaving the essential oil in the still.

RIPENING, PRESERVATION, ETC.

Finally the scent of the extract is to be made tenacious and of agreeable character. The extracts, therefore, are allowed to keep undisturbed in closely sealed vessel in a place not too warm and unexposed to the direct action of sunlight. This greatly ripens the preparation, improves its quality and makes it clearer by the deposition of sediments in solution. To make the fixation complete the volatile portions of the perfumes are to be fixed by less evanescent bodies. The alcohol, when in use, produces a disagreeable smell which is also to be remedied.

SECTION TWO
ESSENTIAL EXTRACTS

CHAPTER VI

FLORAL OILS

The preparation of floral oils constitutes by itself a big industry distinctly of Indian origin, and their manufacture can easily be traced to many centuries ago. To this day a flourishing industry centres round Jaunpur, Ghazipur, Lucknow, Delhi and other celebrated parts of Northern India.

SELECTION OF SITE

Flowers play an important part in the manufacture of floral oils. It may be noticed by the common observer that the industry thrives in places where finest flowers abound and are available in plenty for treatment and manufacture. A place without this natural advantage and where flower cultivation is not in systematic progress, can hardly prove to be the nursery of a successful floral oil industry. There are many places in India where the finest flowers can be propagated or grown but are allowed to go to waste, and it is at these places that a safe industry can be founded to the great benefit of the country.

RAW MATERIALS

Any flower with a decent smell can be utilised for the manufacture of floral oils. But the flowers most employed are bela, chameli, henna, jasmine, gandharaj, kamini, etc., etc., and the floral oils obtained from these flowers are most relished and appeal to the general taste.

The common vehicle in the preparation of floral oils is sesamum oil, though sometimes it is replaced by olive oil. Sesamum oil, however, seems to be the most suited basis for the manufacture of floral oils; for, this by itself possesses several meritorious properties. It keeps the hair soft and the brain cool. Over and above this, the oil has got fixative properties which enable it to bind down the fragrance of the flowers for a long time to come, even on exposure to air or on being washed with water at the time of bathing.

TREATMENT OF THE INGREDIENTS

In preparing the floral oils, only the full-blown flowers should be selected. These should be as fresh as possible. Special notice is to be taken of the fact that the flowers should be all of the same standard quality and of the same colour, specially in the case of rose. Before being treated the flowers should also be freed from dust and earth and the stalks should also be removed from them without unduly pressing the petals.

As regards sesamum oil, only the best refined oils should be used for making floral oils. Special notice need be taken of the fact that only earthern, glass, chinaclay, porcelain, enamelled ware and aluminium utensils are to be used during manipulations. No iron, copper or brazen wares should be employed, for, these are very likely to react on the oil.

There are several methods of extracting the odoriferous principles from the flowers though the underlying principles in each case is either infusion, digestion or maceration or a combination of them. The general processes of manufacturing floral oils are put below.

MANUFACTURE BY MACERATION

The fresh scented flowers are freed from stalks and are steeped in about double their weight of sesamum oil contained in a wide-mouthed bottle or jar, preferably of glass. The ingredients are then put in the sun, taking care to cover up the mouth of the vessel so that no dust or sand can enter the jar. The jar is continually kept in the sun and sometimes in the dew at night for a considerable period of time which may vary from a week to a month. The oil is then filtered through a piece of flannel or sometimes through cloth and the filtrate is collected. Care should be exercised that the flowers do not get mashed during the process. It is evident that some oil adheres to the surface of the exhausted flowers; a successful manufacturer however does not allow this oil to go to waste. With this object in view the flowers are put in a big glass funnel having a small orifice to allow the settling oil to drip. The dripping oil is carefully collected and mixed with the previously filtered oil. The sesamum oil can thus be made to imbibe the odour of the flowers, yielding the floral oils of commerce. The oil should then be put in vessels having mouths closed tightly with stoppers to avoid contact with air.

CONCENTRATING THE PREPARATIONS

But on many occasions it will be found that the sesamum oil is not sufficiently odorous and can be made to absorb further odour. In such cases the oil is charged with a fresh lot of new-blown flowers freed from stalks. The whole is then placed in an aluminium pan, covered up and heated on the water bath for about half an hour. The pan is set aside for 24 hours in an undisturbed position and the oil is then strained. The soaked flowers are placed on a funnel and allowed to drip, and the oil is collected below. The waste flowers are then thrown away. The two oils are then mixed and filtered once again. Sometimes the filtered oil is given a third charge of flowers and the same operation is repeated before the process is brought to a close.

HASTENING THE PROCESS

It will be observed that the above method to be successful requires strong sunlight for a considerable time, moreover the complete process requires a pretty long time. When, however, the operations are required to be completed within a short measure of time, the flowers are infused in about double their quantity of sesamum oil and instead of putting the two ingredients in the sun continually for a number of days, they are put in an aluminium pan, covered up and heated on water bath for half an hour, and then set aside for 24 hours. The oil is strained and the exhausted flowers are thrown away after the collection of the adhering oils in a manner described above. When the final product is desired to be of excellent quality the operation is repeated 7 or 8 times.

In lieu of repeated boiling on water bath, sometimes the filtered oil after a single heating on water bath and collection, is given a further charge of fresh flowers and the whole is set aside for a number of days in the sun after closing the mouth of the vessel tightly.

TIER SYSTEM

A third method is sometimes adopted. Several pieces of white cotton cloth are soaked in sesamum or olive oil and are then wrung out. The cotton cloth thus moistened is spread at the bottom of a suitable vessel and a quantity of flower is laid over it. This layer of flower is then covered up by a second piece of cloth previously wetted and fresh flowers are again laid over it. This layer in its turn is covered up by a third cotton cloth. A tier of flowers may thus be made with seven or eight layers of flowers, each separated by moistened cotton cloths. Finally a quantity of oil is poured on the top of the tier. Generally the oil should be of double the weight of the flowers taken. The whole is then set aside for a number of days; the oil is then strained and collected. The process is repeated several times when oils of excellent quality are required.

ANOTHER TIER ARRANGEMENT

Essentially the same principle of extraction of the floral oils may be applied in another manner by substituting raw cotton in place of the cotton cloth. In a big-sized aluminium vessel, fresh flowers are first strewn over in a layer and these are then covered over thoroughly by loose and clean cotton. Then sesamum oil equalling the weight of the flowers taken is poured on the flowers. Fresh flowers are again laid out in the same manner and are entirely covered over thickly by loose cotton; and sesamum oil is again poured on the cleaned cotton. Several layers of flowers, cotton and oil are arranged in this manner. Sometimes as many as eight are made. Then the vessel is placed in the sun for a number of days after its mouth is closed duly. Finally the cotton and the flowers are pressed, together to obtain the oil.

The cotton pads are not thrown away. Fresh lots of flowers are strewn in a vessel, then a part of the wet cotton is laid over the flowers and a part of the above extracted oil is poured on the layer. As many as eight layers are arranged in this way and then the whole is placed in the sun after closing the mouth. The cotton and flowers are next extracted as before. This operation is generally repeated 5 or 6 times in order to obtain a good quality oil.

OIL DIRECT FROM THE SEEDS

Sesamum seeds are often employed in place of the sesamum oil for making the floral oils. In such cases, the fresh flowers are strewn over in a layer and are thoroughly covered by a layer of sesamum seeds. On the layer thus formed sesamum oil is then poured. The vessel is then placed in the sun for a certain number of days. It must however be covered up during the process of sunning. Then the exhausted flowers are replaced by fresh flowers and then the operation is repeated over again several times. Finally the mixture of sesamum seeds and oils is cold pressed in *ghanies* or oil mills, to yield a high class oil with pleasing odour.

The sesamum seeds are sometimes ground and brayed on a muller with a roller and the paste is then applied to the flowers. These may be put in the sun and then boiled with sesamum oil over a water bath. Or, the paste may be put in the sesamum oil and flowers may then be steeped in the mixture and heated on a water bath. The whole mass is then strained and the oil is obtained, which may be similarly treated several times for high quality products.

RECIPES

With these observations we give a number of recipes which may be adopted with slight modifications for the preparation of other floral oils.

BELA OIL

Procedure: Take 1 sr. fresh *Bela* flowers and 2½ srs. of sesamum oil. Put the two together into a wide-mouthed bottle; close it up tightly and place for seven days in the sun and in the dew at night.

Then strain through a flannel taking care that the flowers are not mashed. Put the flowers on a funnel and allow to drip. Collect the oil in an aluminium vessel and steep into it another lot of 1 seer of flowers, heat the vessel on the water bath for an hour and set aside for 24 hours. Now filter the oil, steep into it a third lot of 1 seer flowers and heat on the water bath for half an hour.

Finally filter. In this way a highly concentrated oil will be obtained.

JASMINE OIL

Procedure: Take several pieces of clean and white cotton cloth; soak them in olive oil, rasp and wring out. Spread a piece of the cloth thus wetted at the bottom of a suitable vessel and lay out a quantity of Jasmine flowers on it. Cover it up with a second piece of cotton cloth and again lay out flowers over it. Cover it with a third piece of cotton cloth. Now pour sesamum oil on the top layer. The quantity of the oil should be double that of flowers. Set aside for 24 hours. Then press the soaked flowers and collect the oil. Repeat the process seven times. Finally strain and squeeze the oil and bottle.

CHAMELI OIL

Procedure: Take 1 sr. *Chameli* flower and 1 sr. sesamum. Lay out the flowers in an aluminium vessel and pour 1 seer sesamum oil; close up the mouth of the vessel and place it in the sun for 3 days. Now pick out the exhausted flowers and put in a fresh lot of 1 sr. flowers into it. Cover the mouth again and place in the sun for 7 days, after which period pick out the exhausted flowers and put a third lot of 1 sr. flowers into the oil. Cover the mouth and place in the sun again for 15 days. Now finally pick out the exhausted flowers and express the mixture of sesamum seeds and oil to obtain a nicely scented oil.

CHAMPAKA OIL

Procedure: Put 200 *Champaka* flowers in a jar and pour 2½ srs. sesamum oil into it. Close up the mouth and place in the sun for 7 days and in the dew at night. Then press out the oil and give a fresh charge of flowers. This process may be repeated eight times when a highly scented oil will be obtained.

KANTALI CHAMPAKA OIL

Procedure: Take 100 fresh *Kantali Champaka* flowers and 1½ srs. good olive oil. Put the two together into an aluminium pot, cover up and heat in the water bath for half an hour. Remove the vessel and set aside for 24 hours. Strain through a flannel and put in a bottle. Now take the oil again in the vessel, put in a fresh lot of 100 flowers, heat again for half an hour and set aside for 24 hours. Press out the oil, collect it in the vessel, put in a third lot of 100 flowers, heat for half an hour and set aside for 24 hours. Finally strain and bottle. The soaked flowers may be squeezed to yield oil.

JAHURI CHAMPAKA OIL

Procedure: Take ½ seer newly blown *Jahuri Champaka* flowers and 10 srs. almond oil. Reject the green portion and put them in a bottle. Pour in the oil and place in the sun for 15 days and in the dew at night. Then strain the oil and steep in it another lot of $1/_2$ sr. fresh flowers, close up the mouth and place in the sun for 15 days. Finally press the oil, filter and bottle.

DOLAN CHAMPAKA OIL

Procedure: Take 1 sr. of *Nageswar Champakas* from stalks and 1 sr. sesamum oil into a wide-mouthed bottle and place for 2 days in the sun and in the dew at night. Strain the oil and put it again in the bottle, steep a fresh lot of $1/_2$ sr. flowers; set aside for 24 hours and strain the oil. Put in a third lot of flowers in the oil; set aside for 24 hours and finally press out the oil, filter and bottle.

NAGESWAR CHAMPAKA OIL

Procedure: Take 1 sr. of *Nageswar Champakas* free from stalks and 1 sr. sesamum oil into a wide-mouthed bottle and place for 2 days in the sun and in the dew at night. Strain the oil and put it again in the bottle, steep a fresh lot of $\frac{1}{2}$ sr. flowers; set aside for 24 hours and strain the oil. Put in a third lot of flowers in the oil; set aside for 24 hours and finally press out the oil, filter and bottle.

HENNA OIL

Procedure: Take 2½ srs. sesamum oil in an aluminium vessel, cover up and heat on a water bath for an hour. Then put 1 sr. *Mehndi* flowers into it and set aside for 24 hours. Then press the oil from the flowers. Take the pressed oil in the vessel and heat it again on the water bath for half an hour. Now steep into this oil a fresh lot of 1 sr. flowers, set aside for 24 hours and then press out the oil. Put the oil in a wide-mouthed bottle; steep in it $1\ 1/_2$ srs. flowers, cork it air-tight and place the bottle in the sun for a fortnight. Finally filter the oil through a piece of flannel and mix the drippings with the original oil.

GUL HENNA OIL

Procedure: Take 1 sr. *Mehndi* flowers, ½ ch. saffron and ¼ sr. sesamum. First bray the saffron and sesamum together into a fine paste, on a stone with a muller. Now pour into the paste 1½ srs. of sesamum oil. Soak the flowers into the mixture. Cover up and heat on the water bath for half an hour. Set aside the vessel for 24 hours. Strain the whole mass through a flannel, squeezing it to press the oil. Put the pressed oil in a wide-mouthed bottle and steep in it another lot of 1 sr. flowers. Place the bottle in the sun for 20 days. Finally strain through a flannel and store in jars.

MUSK HENNA OIL

Procedure: Take 2 seers of *Mehndi* flowers 2½ srs. of sesamum oil and $1/_8$ tollah of musk. Macerate the musk in a stone mortar in 1 ch. of oil thoroughly. Put the colate in an aluminium vessel with the flowers and heat it on the water bath for an hour. Then put the oil in a wide-mouthed vessel, close up the mouth tightly and place it for seven days in the sun and in the dew at night. Finally strain through a flannel and store in bottles or jars.

JANTI OIL

Procedure: Take 1 seer of dry *Janti* flowers and add 1 seer olive oil. Put the two together into a bottle and place in the sun for a month. After that press the oil and collect it in an aluminium vessel. Steep into it a second lot of 1 sr. fresh flowers. Cover up and heat on the water bath for 24 hours.

MALLIKA OIL

Procedure: Take 2½ srs. *Mallika* flowers and 2 srs. of sesamum oil. Put the two together into a wide-mouthed bottle and close air-tight. Place the bottle in the sun for a month. Then strain through a piece of flannel. Put the soaked flowers in a funnel and allow to drip. Mix the two oils together.

TUBEROSE OIL

Procedure: Take 3 srs. pure olive oil and 1½ srs. tuberoses. Put the two together in an aluminium vessel. Cover up and heat on the water bath for half an hour. Remove, set aside for 24 hours, and press gently to squeeze out the oil. Collect it in a wide-mouthed bottle and steep in the oil another lot of 2 srs. flowers. Close air-tight and set aside for a month. Finally express the oil, filter it and bottle.

ROSE OIL

Procedure: Take ½ sr. of sesamum oil in a suitable vessel and throw into it $1/_8$ sr. petals of fresh roses of the same colour. Cover up and heat on the water bath for half an hour. Set the vessel aside for 24 hours. Pour out on a piece of clean cloth and wring to press out the whole oil. Again steep a fresh lot of $1/_2$ sr. rose petals in the expressed oil and follow the above directions. It the process be repeated 7 or 8 times, the final product will be of excellent quality and command high price.

BAKUL OIL

Procedure: Take 1 sr. *Bakul flowers* and 1 sr. sesamum oil. Put the two together into a jar, close up the mouth and put it in the sun for a month. Then express the oil.

KETAKI OIL

Procedure: Take 1 sr. pollen of *Ketaki* flowers, ½ sr. minced petals (white and tender), and 2 srs. of sesamum oil. Put these ingredients together in a jar, close up the mouth and place it for a month in the sun and in the dew at night. Then pour out into a cloth and express the oil. Finally filter and bottle.

KAMINI OIL

Procedure: Take 2 srs. of *Kamini* flowers (free from stalks) and 4 srs. of sesamum oil together in an aluminium pan and cover up and heat on a water bath for half an hour. Then pour the mixture in a wide-mouthed bottle, cork it tight and place in the sun continually for 15 days. Finally strain through a piece of flannel, and put the oil in air-tight bottles.

LEMON FLOWER OIL

Procedure: Take 1 seer fresh *Lemon* flowers, free them from stalks; also take 2½ srs. of sesamum oil; put the two together in a jar and place in the sun continually for a month. Then strain the mixture and drain the flowers. Now take another seer of fresh flowers and put them in the above filtered oil. Put the mixture in a pan, cover up and heat on the water bath for half an hour. Set the pan aside for 24 hours and then strain the oil.

GANDHARAJ OIL

Procedure: Grind thoroughly 2½ srs. of sesamum and mix with the paste 2½ srs. of *Gandharaj* flowers. Put the mixture in a suitable vessel, cover up and place in the sun for 7 days. Then mix 2 srs. sesamum oil into it and heat the mixture on the water bath for one hour. Cover up and set aside for 24 hours. Then strain and put the oil in a bottle. Squeeze the soaked flowers and mix the oil so obtained with the above. Finally filter the whole quantity of oil.

MADHUMALATI OIL

Procedure: Procure 1 sr. *Madhumalati* flowers free from stalk and 1 sr. sesamum oil. Take a big-sized aluminium vessel and strew at its bottom 2 ch. flowers. Lay out over them loose cleaned cotton thickly so as to cover thoroughly. Pour on the cotton 2 ch. oil and strew another layer of flowers. Lay out on it another pad of cotton, pour 2 ch. oil on it and strew flowers. Repeat in this way to make 8 layers. Close up the mouth of the vessel and place in the sun for 24 hours. Now press the cotton and flowers together to obtain the oil.

Do not throw away the cotton pads. Take a fresh lot of flowers; strew a quantity at the bottom of the vessel; lay on it the wet cotton; pour the above extracted oil and arrange in 8 layers. Place in the sun for 24 hours and press the cotton and flowers as before. If this process be repeated for 5 times, an oil of good quality will be obtained.

KHUS OIL

Procedure: Take 2 srs. *Khus* root and 1 sr. sesamum; grind the two together into a paste on a clean stone slab with a muller. If the materials are too dry they may be moistened with a little sesamum oil. Put the paste in a jar, pour into it 2 srs. of sesamum oil and bury the vessel in the earth for one month. The mouth of the jar should be covered with a lid and plastered with mud. After the lapse of the period, bring up and extract the oil to the last drop by pressing hard. Collect the oil in a wide-mouthed vessel. Now take another seer of *Khus*, clean it thoroughly from dirt, and pound it finely in a *dhenki* (country-made rice huller) or in an iron mortar and pestle. Throw the powder thus obtained into the oil already expressed; cover up the mouth of the bottle, place in the sun for 16 days. Finally extract the oil by pressing hard.

LOTUS OIL

Procedure: Procure 5 srs. of white petals of *Lotus* and 5 srs. seasamum oil. Put the two together into a vessel and heat on the water bath for an hour. Remove and set aside for 24 hours. The operations should be carried on under cover. Extract the oil by pressing the soaked petals. Again put $2\,^1/_2$ srs. petals in the oil; heat on the water bath for half an hour. Set aside for 24 hours and extract the oil by pressing. Steep a third lot of 1 sr. flowers in the extracted oil, heat on the water bath for half an hour, set aside for 24 hours and extract the oil. Steep again and place in the sun for 15 days. Extract the oil by pressing; filter and bottle.

STORING

After the preparation of the floral oils, these are stored carefully in vases in cool but not damp places. On many occasions they are stored in pot-bellied vessels made of the membranes from the intestines of sheep, goat, etc. These vessels can be transported from one place to another as they are immune from breakage or leakage, very common in cases of glass or earthen vessels. Apart from the advantages of transport, these vessels are considered to be the best so far as the keeping quality of the oils is concerned. In fact in centres of floral oil manufacture these vessels are much in vogue and are recommended strongly for packing oils.

CHAPTER VII

ESSENTIAL OILS

The preparation of essential oils does not fall directly within the scope of perfumes and cosmetics but their wide application in the manufacture of various perfumery and their valuable medicinal and other properties entitle them to greater attention than hitherto paid to them.

The production of essential oils in India is carried out, literally speaking, from north to south, with important centres of production in Punjab, United Provinces, Central Provinces, Orissa, the Nilgiris, Mysore and Travancore. The important oils apart from the Indian attars, are as follows:

(a) Eucalyptus oil.
(b) Gingergrass oil.
(c) Khus oil.
(d) Lemon Grass oil.
(e) Linaloe oil.
(f) Palmarosa oil.
(g) Rose oil.
(h) Sandalwood oil.
(i) Turpentine oil.

Small quantities of other oils are also produced in India but there is no proper organised effort and the production is thus spasmodic. A beginning has been made to produce citrus oils on a commercial scale in the Punjab and in the Bombay Presidency and of ajwan oil at Indore. Similarly at Kuppam in South India efforts are being made to distil patchouli oil from imported Singapore leaves whilst spasmodic production of geranium oil is reported at Yercaud on the Sheveroy Hills and of wormwood and camphor oil in the Nilgiris. In Mangalore cinnamon oil and in Orissa salresin oil are being produced by crude methods. Any figures of production of these oils are not however available.

ODORIFEROUS ELEMENTS

There is a wide range of odoriferous materials available in India and elsewhere. Of course the flowers are the most noted illustration, but, besides these, there are substances like cinnamon, cloves, cardamom, lime, citrus, lemon, sandalwood, almond etc., etc., which possess peculiar odours of their own, primarily due to the presence of some essential principles in their structure. These may be extracted, and then sold as raw materials for perfumery and for medicine also.

PRELIMINARY TREATMENT

The general principle of manufacture is simple to understand, but great care should be exercised in handling the operations, if high quality of the final product is to be attained. All the materials used for extraction should be of the best type, fresh, undamaged and not perforated by worms and insects. The materials are first shelled and bruised carefully, crushed or cut into pieces and sometimes even pounded or made into paste by braying with a muller on a stone slab as preliminary steps to the manufacture of essential oils. In fact the raw materials should be in a state to be easily permeated by the perfume-bearing vehicle. The materials should also be freed from all dust or dirt. Perfect cleanliness should be observed during all operations. These factors decide the amount of essential oil that can be secured from the stuff.

PROCESSES OF MANUFACTURE

The following general methods are adopted for the manufacture of essential oils:

(a) Maceration.
(b) Distillation.
(c) Expression.
(d) Enfleurage.
(e) Solvent extraction.

BY MACERATION

The general method adopted is to steep the raw materials in olive or sesamum oil in an enamelled vessel or aluminium vessel. Employ no utensils that are liable to react on the oil. Glass, earthenware or porcelain utensils are generally used. The mouth of the vessel should then be covered up carefully to prevent the admission of dust and dirt. In case of substances that yield essential oils easily, without heat, the whole may be placed in the sun for a number of days. Heating in such cases would destroy the delicate essential oil. But when the articles are not of tender variety, but are hard and stiff by nature, simply placing in the sun would not be found sufficient. In such cases the extraction should be completed by the aid of moderate heat. It should be noted that the less an essential oil is heated, the better is its quality. The vessel, therefore, should not be heated, on a direct oven but on water bath so that the heating operation may continue slowly without causing the evaporation of the volatile essential oil or any deterioration in the final product. Generally, the heating need not be continued for more than half an hour. The vessel is allowed to remain undisturbed for a full day and finally the oil is pressed out or strained and the exhausted materials are thrown out.

Exhaustion of Oil-Bearing Sources

Particular notice should be taken that the raw materials after the sunning or boiling operations are fully washed out and no essential principle is allowed to run to waste. Upon this would materially depend the success of the manufacturers. The duration of sunning or of heating should always be so adjusted that the raw materials yield up the essential contents in full or in so far as possible without injuring the quality of the stuff produced.

Concentration of the Oil

The oil thus prepared will often be found to contain not as much essential oil as it can imbibe under ordinary conditions and it should be always the endeavour of the manufacturers that the essential oil prepared is surcharged with the maximum amount of the essential principle it is capable of containing. The quality of the oil is greatly dependent upon this factor and it is the concentrated preparations that command the market and fetch high prices as well.

To attain a high concentration the oil previously obtained is further treated with a fresh lot of the raw materials and the same operations are undergone in full, though the processes of extraction described here are sometimes followed alternately as will be evident from a study of the following recipes. This, however, does not finish the operation and the process is repeated over and over again to get the best results.

Collecting the Oil

A novel method of collecting the oil is adopted sometimes during the process of extraction. The raw materials after being finely bruised are put in a porous vessel and are covered over with sesamum or olive oil and put in strong sunlight. The vessel is put under the hole to collect the dripping oil which is fairly imbibed with the essential matters. The oil may again be poured over the raw materials for further extraction till these are fully exhausted.

The pressing out of the oil requires special care and unless this is done properly there are chances of great losses which should by no means be allowed to go undetected, if the industry is to be based on a sound footing. All measures should be adopted to get the maximum quantity of the oil. When the sunning or heating operations are finished, the oil should be strained out and the remainder should be squeezed forcibly to secure all the oil. The whole may also be allowed to drip through a fine clean cloth so that the oil may ooze out slowly, or a device as mentioned above may also be found profitable and practicable too.

BY DISTILLATION

Essential oils are also procured by distilling the odoriferous substances along with water. For this purpose the oil bearing substance is introduced into a still, water is poured upon it, and heat being applied, the oil is volatilised by the aid of watery vapour at the temperature of 212°F, though when alone it would probably not distil over unless the heat were 100°F more. The mixed vapours which pass over, condense and fall as a milky looking liquid into the receiver. This separates after a time into two portions, one of which is a solution of a part of the newly eliminated oil in water and the other is the oil itself which can then be collected. Roshagrass, lemon grass, camphor, eucalyptus, peppermint, rose, *ketaki*, sandal, orange, cloves, cinnamon, cardamom, citronella grass, and many oil bearing substances may be distilled in this way.

The Report of the Essential Oil Committee (Exploratory) by P.A. Narialwala and J.M. Rakshit writes that distillation process is the most widely used throughout the world. This system is found to be still prevalent in almost all the centres in India producing essential oils. This mehtod is however, a crude method as it affects both the quality and the yield of the oils. On the other hand, a better method would be distillation by steam since it is quicker in operation and gives a better yield and quality of oil and enables the operation to be controlled in a scientific manner. The difficulty of setting up steam distillation units in inaccessable places where aromatic plants grow has largely contributed to the Indian distillers still resorting to the old water distillation method because of its being the cheapest and most simple for conducting the operation. It is time that the essential oil manufacturers devote some thought on the problem of improving the distilling methods practised in India. A small distilling aparatus which may be used under open fire gives better results than the old water distillation method. The water distillation method is suitable for producing oil from roots, grasses, leaves and some varieties of flowers; it is, therefore, the most popular and universal method employed for the extraction of essential oils.

BY EXPRESSION

In a few instances the essential oils are obtained by direct expression of rinds and fruits, as in the case of lemons, oranges, etc., but in these cases the expressed oils are not equal to the products obtained by distillation. These are not so white, nor do they keep so well.

This method is utilised, and has been developed particularly like Italy, for the expression of delicate essential oils from the peels of citrus fruits like oranges, lemons, etc. The peels are pressed over sponges from which the absorbed oil is recovered by squeezing with hand. It is no doubt possible to extract the essential oil from citrus peels by steam distillation, but the oil has been found to lack the freshness of aroma which is usually associated with hand pressed oils which fetch a better price.

ENFLEURAGE

This method according to the Report referred to above is employed for extracting the oil from flowers like jasmine, tuberoses, etc., by mixing the flower with a pure fat on specially devised trays. The fat absorbs the odoriferous bodies present in the flowers and when it is saturated with the perfumes present in the flowers it is shaken with alcohol which dissolves the perfume but not the fat.

This method of extraction was known as practised in India many centuries ago and has been mentioned in "Ain-i-Akbari." It is practised in India even to-day for the production of scented oils which are generally made from sesamum seeds. Wetted sesamum seed are placed in alternate layers with the flowers, and are left over for 12 to 18 hours; the seeds are then crushed in a mill and the scented oil is obtained.

The Indian method of enfleurage is however different from the European method where the extract is obtained in a solid form known as "concrete" which consists of the flower oil in solution in natural waxes present in the flowers. From the 'concrete' the natural flowers oil, often called the 'absolute' is separated by suitable solvents. The "concretes" and the "absolutes" obtained by the enfleurage method are very expensive but are invaluable in the blending of high quality perfumes as well as synthetic flower oils.

SOLVENT EXTRACTION

This process* is generally used in recovering oils having a delicate flowery note, which may ordinarily be destroyed under steam distillation. The solvent commonly employed is petroleum ether of low boiling point. The solvent is boiled in a separate vessel, and the vapours are allowed to enter a rotary drum in which baskets containing the flowers to be extracted are fitted; these baskets are pierced so that the vapours pass freely through the flowers as well as from one basket to another; by keeping the drum in rotation, fresh solvent comes at regular intervals in contact with the flowers.

There is also another method in which the solvent is allowed to pass through a series of vessels, and extraction is carried out

---
* Taken from Report on Essential Oil.

by the counter current system in which fresh solvent is allowed to pass over flowers which has already given up most of their perfume by previous extraction. The saturated solvent is evaporated and an "absolute" of the flower perfume is obtained. Although the method has greatly improved lately and has partly replaced the enfleurage method, on account of its rapidity of execution, the quality of "absolute" obtained by the enfleurage method is still considered to be far superior. In fact both the methods are coupled in modern factories in the West and the flowers used in the enfleurage method are subsequently treated by volatile solvents for thorough extraction of odoriferous materials which had no time to dissolve in the fat. This method is not in use in India now.

ABSOLUTES

The manufacture of pure natural oils of flowers or "absolutes" of jasmine, moghra, bokul, etc., is practically unknown in India, but the attars of these and other flowers are produced at Kanauj and Ghazipur, where the method of manufacture consists of heating the flowers mixed with water under an open fire in a copper vessel which is connected to a pot containing sandalwood oil into which the vapours are allowed to condense. After the separation of water, the mixture of sandalwood oil and natural flower oil constitute the attar of India, and the quality of an attar is determined by the concentration of natural flower oil in it.

PRESERVATION

Essential oils must be guarded from the action of light and air. Light turns the oils darker and sometimes blackens the oils. The oxygen from air acts on some essential oils, making them viscid. These oils should be bottled in clean and dry glass stoppered bottle and stored in a dark place. Addition of $1/2$ to 1 per cent absolute alcohol to the essential oils preserves the same well.

PROPERTIES

Finally it should be known that some of the essential oils are colourless while others are green or dark brown in colour. As a general rule the essential oils are lighter than water though there are exceptions to the rule as in the case of cinnamon oil.

The oils are also liable to oxidation if exposed to air; hence they are to be carefully and tightly packed in phials filled to the top and sealed if necessary to prevent contact with air and consequent decomposition. Ground glass stoppers are mostly used to close the mouth air-tight. The phials should preferably be placed in the dark and in a cool, not damp place.

A few recipes are given below with notes culled from the Report of the Essential Oil Committee (Exploratory) by P.A. Narialwala and J.N. Rakshit:

AJWAN OIL

Ajwan oil is obtained from the Ajwan seeds and has use in the pharmaceutical and perfumery industry. This oil is produced at present on a commercial scale at Rao in Indore state; a little of it is also produced in the United Provinces. In Indore the oil is produced by steam distillation. It is said that one ton of seed yields about 56 lbs. of oil. From the oil is also recovered thymol crystals, after the extraction of which the residue is sold under a new trade name of "Thymoil."

AMLA OIL

I

Procedure: Take 2½ seers sesamum brayed to a paste, 5 seers emblic myrobalan free from seeds and bruised, and 10 seers sesamum oil. Put the three ingredients together in an iron vessel and place in the sun for one month. Strain out only 5 seers of the soaking oil and put in a fresh lot of 5 seers sesamum oil. Leave aside for one month; strain out again 5 seers of oil and put in a third and fresh lot of 5 seers of oil. Repeat the operation for 6 months. Then strain the whole of the oil and mix together the former quantities. Put in a covered vessel.

Amla oil prepared in this way serves as a good hair dye. Smear the head with it every day half an hour before bath. The hair will be dyed black and no grey hair will be noticeable.

II

Procedure: Take 4 srs. of raw and good sesamum oil and 4 srs. cleaned and crushed emblic myrobalans. First steep the myrobalans in water for 24 hours; pound them thoroughly and dissolve in 16 srs. of water. Then put the oil in an iron pan and apply moderate heat. When the oil has bubbled for some time and the froth has subsided, remove the pan some distance away from the oven. Now take a ladle with a long handle, fill it with the above decoction of myrobalan and sprinkle the same on the hot oil. This should be done from a distance, taking every precaution to prevent any accident. Just as the water will be poured on the oil there will be a deafening sound; but the operation should be carried through without any fear. After the whole quantity of the decoction is thus blended with the oil, put the pan on the fire and continue boiling. When the water has evaporated, remove the pan and set it aside with the oil for 7 days. Finally filter and bottle.

ANISEED OIL

Procedure: Take ½ sr. aniseed; pick and dust carefully. Pound and macerate them in ½ sr. good olive oil and put the pulp in a porous iron vessel. Hold a vessel under the hole and place the whole arrangement in bright sunlight. The oil will drip. When it is exhausted put the oil in a stoppered phial.

CAMPHOR OIL

Camphor oil is produced from camphor trees (Variety Laurus Camphora) at Coonoor. On distillation of the leaves, solid camphor and camphor oil are obtained. About 500 lbs. of camphor and 100 lbs. of camphor oil are produced per annum at Coonoor. The percentage of camphor in the oil obtained from different portions of the tree by steam distillation is as follows:

Green leaves 40.6 per cent; leaves 43.0 per cent; dry leaves 30.5 per cent; twigs from 20 to 35.5 per cent; branches from 0 to 12 per cent; roots from 24.0 to 28.7 per cent; stumps from 17.5 to 25 per cent.

Camphor oil is now almost entirely produced in Japan. Camphor trees take several years to grow and to be of benefit for the production of camphor and camphor oil. Due to the commercial importance of these products attempts should be made to grow camphor trees on a large scale in various parts of India.

It may be mentioned here that camphor trees can be successfully cultivated in all parts of India with an annual rainfall of 40 inches and over and a satisfactory yield of oil, rich in camphor, can be obtained from the leaves.

CINNAMON OIL

Procedure: Take 2 ch. of pounded cinnamon and one seer good olive oil; put the two together in a vessel and close it up. Heat on the water bath for half an hour. Leave aside for 24 hours and then squeeze out the oil. Put the oil again into the same vessel and steep in it 2 ch. pounded cinnamon. Cover the mouth of the vessel and heat on the water bath for half an hour. Leave aside for 24 hours and then squeeze out the oil. For the third time put the oil into the same vessel and steep in it 2 ch. pounded cinnamon. Heat on the water bath for half and hour. Leave aside for 24 hours. Finally strain and bottle in a stoppered phial.

Mention may be made in this connection that cinnamon oil is distilled by a few firms in Mangalore by crude methods from the cinnamon bark as well as the leaves of the cinnamon trees which grow abundantly in Malabar and South Canara. The oils from the leaves and the bark differ in their chemical constituents, the oil from the bark being more valuable, though both the oils are of considerable importance in pharmaceutical industry, in the flavouring of the foods, and manufacture of aromatic chemicals. The oil from the bark, also known as Cassia Oil, yields the important aromatic Cinnamic Aldehyde whilst the leaf oil is a source of Eugenol. In view of the fact that cinnamon trees thrive well in India the development of the cinnamon oil industry from the bark as well as the leaf is an immediate possibility.

CITRUS OILS

Citrus oils find an immediate sale in India itself. The manufacture of the oils other than lime was undertaken after considerable research at the Chemical Laboratories of the Punjab University particularly. The manufacture of lime oils was also undertaken after a careful investigation of the problem by the Department of Industries, Bombay. The lime tree is indigenous to India and grows throughout the country. In Bombay Presidency the area under cultivation is estimated to be 1,200 acres.

The lime oil is used as a flavouring material for food and beverages and there is demand for it both in Europe as well as in the United States. The oil is distilled by steam from the rinds and juice of the fruits and it is reported that on an average about 2 per cent of oil is recovered.

In India, oranges, sweet limes, lemons, etc., grow in a number of places. The Central Provinces, the Punjab, the North Western Provinces, the Khasi Hills, in Assam, the Sheveroys and the Wynads on the Western Ghats, the Bamra State in Orissa and Coorg are important centres of cultivation of citrus trees. The following varieties of citrus plants are recorded as being grown in India.

1. Citrus Bigaradia Risso (Bitter Orange).
2. Citrus Aurantium Linn (Sweet Orange 'Narangi').
3. Citrus Nobilis Lour (Mandarin or Maltese Orange).
4. Citrus Decumana Linn (Paradise apple— 'Batabi' Limbu).
5. Citrus Medica Linn (The Citron).
6. Citrus Limonum (Limon—'Kaghzi').
7. Citrus Lemetta (Sweet Lime—'Mitha Limbu').
8. Citrus Acids (Sour Lime—'Limbu').

The varieties of essential oils that can be obtained from either the peels, the flowers or the leaves of each variety are given below in serial order:

1. Petit grain oil from the leaves of the bitter orange and bitter orange oil from fruits.
2. Oil of sweet orange from leaves, of the Narangi variety, oils of Neroli Portugal from flowers, and oil of sweet orange from fruits.
3. Oil of Mandarin leaves from leaves of Maltese Orange and oil of Mandarin from fruits.
4. Grape fruit oil from fruits of the Batabi limbu.
5. Oil of linnette leaves from leaves of the Citron and oil of citrus from fruits.
6. Oil of lemon from fruits of the Kaghzi limbu.
7. Oil of limmette flowers from flowers of sweet lime and oil of limmette from fruits.
8. Oil of lime from fruits of sour limes.

The citrus oils are indispensible in the manufacture of fine perfumery, but their largest use is as a flavouring material in foods, confectionery, aerated waters and tobacco. At present in all the citrus pantations in India a considerable quantity of fruits is allowed to rot and go waste. If an attempt was made to recover the oil from the peels of those wasted fruits a considerable additional income would accrue to the plantations. The extraction of true oils from the peel is closely connected with the utilisation of the wasted fruit in the manufacture of marmalades, fruit juices, syrups, etc. Considerable scope, therefore, exists in the development of this industry. Steps should, therefore, be taken to develop the manufacture of citrus oils, citric acid and pectin at the orange and lemon plantations in India so that not only new industries but new wealth may be created in the country.

CLOVES OIL

Procedure: Take one seer bruised cloves and macerate the same in one seer olive oil thoroughly. Put it in a porous iron pot and hold a vessel under the hole. Place the arrangement in hot sun and the oil will drip through the pores. When the oozing ceases, store the oil in a stoppered phial.

CARDAMOM OIL

Procedure: Take 2 ch. bruised seeds of cardamom major and 1 seer of good olive oil. Put the two together in a vessel, cover it up and heat on the water bath for half an hour. Set aside the vessel for 24 hours. Press out the oil and put it again in the vessel. Steep in it another lot of 2 ch. cardamom and heat on the water bath for half an hour. Set aside for 24 hours. Squeeze out the oil once more, steep in it a third lot of 2 ch. cardamom and heat on the water bath for half an hour. Set aside for 24 hours. Then press out the oil thoroughly and store in stoppered phials.

CASSIA OIL

Procedure: Take 4 ch. pounded white cassia leaves and 1 seer good olive oil. Put them in a stoppered phial and close up the mouth neatly. Place it in the strong sun for two months. After that press out the oil and store it in a stoppered phial.

EUCALYPTUS OIL

Eucalyptus oil is obtained from the leaves of the Eucalyptus trees which thrive well on the Nilgiris, the Annamalai and the Palni Hills. The area under cultivation on the Nilgiris is about 2,500 acres whilst the production of oil is nearly 22,000 gallons per annum, equivalent to about 85 tons. The entire production is consumed within the country. It may be interesting to mention here that U.P., Bihar as also certain tracts in Orissa are suitable for eucalyptus plantation. As eucalyptus oil has commercial importance, it would be of benefit to the country if its cultivation on a large scale is undertaken in these areas. Cultivation may be also undertaken of another variety of eucalyptus tree, known as eucalyptus citriodora; the leaves of this variety are reported to be rich in citrionella which is an important aldehyde in perfumery as well as in medicinal industry and is also a starting medium for the manufacture of menthol. The manufacture of eucalyptus oil is conducted by primitive methods as a result of which the purity of the oil varies from batch to batch. It is stated that Indian eucalyptus oil is deficient in the cineol content and, therefore, does not come up to the latest B.P. specifications. The oil contains 60 per cent cineol by volume, which is sufficient for all ordinary use. The Indian oil besides contains no aldehydes, such as valeric, butyric and caprioc aldehydes, the presence of which causes irritation to the throat resulting in coughing and other unpleasant symptoms, which is the case with the Australian oil. Moreover, the yield of oil obtained in the Nilgiris even by primitive methods is reported to be greater than the yield from Australian leaves of the same botanical name.

Procedure: The still used for eucalyptus oil is ordinarily 4 feet high and 2½ feet in diameter made with copper plates at the bottom and iron sheets at the sides. A foot above the bottom of the still is a perforated iron plate over which the leaves are placed so that they will not come in direct contact with the heat. Leaves of mature trees sixteen to seventeen years old are preferred to leaves of younger trees. They are dried for three days after picking before being distilled. Leaves dried in the shade give a greater yield of oil. Before the heating commences the still is filled with water and the required quantity of leaves is placed over the perforated plate. The cover of the still is tightly closed and the vapour is allowed to escape through a pipe into a tub, after first passing through a column of cold water. The condensed vapour contains a large percentage of water.

The oil, being lighter, rises to the surface and the water is allowed to pass through a tap at the bottom of the receptacle. Generally, boiling is continued for 8 hours, the water in the still being maintained at the same level by constant addition as it evaporates. The crude oil thus collected is refined by mixing it with one-sixth the quantity of water and adding a small amount of caustic soda. The mixture is again distilled in a similar but smaller still and the oil is passed through filter papers until it is got rid of all impurities. The material is not directly heated but it is worked up by steam alone. By this means better quality and higher yield of the oil are both secured.

GERANIUM OIL

This oil is distilled from a variety of French geranium probably Pelargonium odoratissima. An acre of geranium rosat yields about 8 lbs. of oil. A wild geranium grows profusely in certain localities on the Nilgiris. The oil is obtained from the leaves and flowers. Geranium oil is an oil of great importance in the perfumery industry as, along with khus and patchouli oils, it forms the body of all good perfume compounds. It is also the basic medium for the manufacture of rhodinol and its esters. The Nilgiris and the Sheveroy Hills are well suited for the cultivation of geranium plants. India can produce a geranium oil of first class quality, which will have not only a market in India but also a large market abroad. Care will have to be taken to see that the right variety of geranium is planted as there are 6 or 7 species of geranium, and certain varieties yield an oil which gives a peppermint note and which may not be acceptable to the perfume industry, which always prefers an oil having a predominant rose odour and without any subsidiary odours.

GINGER GRASS OIL

Ginger grass grows wild in some of the southern districts of Travancore where it is known as "Inchipul." There are two varieties of this grass, one white and the other red, but the oil from both the varieties is similar in respect of odour as well as other qualities. The oil is distilled by crude methods from leaves, grass and flowers on a very small scale. Ginger grass oil is a sweet smelling oil, is different in constituents from lemon grass and palmarosa oil, although it resembles palmarosa oil in odour. The ginger grass oil is, however, rich in Borneol which is of value to the perfumery industry, and it would be, therefore, worthwhile to develop the distillation of ginger grass oil on a larger scale.

KHUS OIL

Khus oil is distilled from the roots of the Khus grass which grows in abundance in widely different parts of India, viz., in Malabar, Orissa, the Punjab, Central Provinces, United Provinces and Bharatpur State. The grass grows wild and no systematic effort has been made to cultivate it or to find out its varieties or which of them will yield the best quality or the highest percentage of oil. The distillation of the roots is carried out by primitive methods on a fairly large scale in Bharatpur and in the United Provinces and to a small extent also in the Punjab and in Orissa. The season for the distillation of oil is from November to February. Khus oil has not only a large market in India itself but has possibilities of an export trade, if an oil of standard quality were to be produced.

LEMON GRASS OIL

Lemon grass grows mainly in the northern districts of Travancore and in a small area in Cochin on an elevation of about 500 feet. Formerly, the grass was also found in central and southern districts of Travancore but this has now ceased. The cutivation of grass is very haphazard and scattered over large areas, some of which are highly inaccessible. Lemon grass is a hardy plant and grows in almost any kind of soil, though it is reported that the more fertile the soil, the more the citral constant in the oil. The life of the grass varies from 6 to 15 years, but 8 to 10 years is the normal productive life. The sowing of the grass takes place towards the end of March or beginning of April and it is reported that the best yield of oil is obtained when the grass is cut during the dry weather. Normally, there are four cuttings in the year at an interval of 6 to 7 weeks starting in May and ending with December. The distillation of the grass is carried out in old-fashioned stills. There is a small consumption of the oil in the country and the bulk of it is exported to Europe and America from Cochin. The solubility of the oil in 70 per cent alcohol is considered by the perfumery trade as a criterion of its purity. The causes of the insolubility are due to the presence of a different grass in the true lemon grass. This grass is like lemon grass in appearance but has a white stem and is usually called the white variety. As it is found to give a higher yield of oil, it is cultivated with true lemon grass, but its harmful effect to the purity of the lemon grass oil has not been realised.

Procedure: Use a steam bath. For heating by steam the most convenient apparatus is a cylindrical vessel 10" in diameter and 15" in height with a conical top. The outside jacket to enclose steam is 14" in diameter and 18" in height with a bottom of three inches height clear for water. The still can hold about 5 lbs. of grass or other similar material. The quantity of oil that can be obtained will depend upon the quality of the material and charges taken per day. It takes about an hour or so for complete distillation of one charge from the time the steam is allowed to pass through.

LEMON RIND OIL, ETC.

Procedure: The distillation of substances, such as, roots, lemon-rinds, Pudina, Kevada, Rose flower, Betelvine leaves, etc., has been carried out by using the above apparatus quite successfully and efficiently and, therefore, it is recommended for the distillation of essential oils.

LINALOE OIL

Linaloe oil is produced from the carpels of Bursera Delpechiana and Bursera Aloexylon though the oil can also be distilled from the leaves as well as the wood. The distillation of the oil is carried out with modern stills under scientific control. Linaloe oil has great possibilities and the extension of linaloe plantation should be encouraged. The important aromatic constituent of linaloe oil is linalol from which it is possible to make linalyl acetate, an important aromatic chemical for the perfumery industry.

LEMON OIL

Procedure: For this purpose citrus lemon of the *pati* variety will be required. Take half a seer of its fresh peels and 1 seer of olive oil. Put the two together in a vessel and heat on the water bath for half an hour. Remove and leave aside for 24 hours. Then press out the oil. Put the oil again in the vessel and steep in it another lot of 4 chhataks of dry peels of lemon grated finely. Close up the mouth of the vessel and place it daily in the sun for one month. Finally strain and bottle in a stoppered phial.

PALMA ROSA OR ROSHA GRASS OIL

This oil is produced from the rosha grass which grows abundantly in the Central Provinces, Bombay Presidency, in some parts of Nizam's Dominions and is also found in Baroda, Gwalior and Indore States. It is unfortunate that no attempt has been made in any of these States to distil the oil. The grass is said to be known in India from ancient times and until recently India was the only source of supply of this oil. Rosha grass is a perennial plant; it grows to a height of about 6 to 8 feet. It is grown from seeds which are generally sown in the month of June before the monsoon starts. In 4 to 5 months the grass is ready for its first cutting and distillation. The oil is distilled from the entire grass including the flower in stalk, the leaves and flowers yielding the most oil. There are eleven varieties of rosha grass of which the "Motia" variety is the best, from the point of view of yield of oil and fragrance; the other varieties yield poor quantity as well as quality of oil. An acre of grass yields 15 to 20 lbs. of oil, severe frost kills the grass and reduces its oil content to as much as 54 per cent. Only the best variety of grass should be grown which is the Motia variety. At present the grass grows in a wild state in the forests and is often inaccessible for exploitation. As India holds an important position in the supply of palma rosa oil, the cultivation of rosha grass should be carried out on most scientific lines.

ORANGE OIL

Procedure: Take one seer of fresh peels of orange and mince them. Take also one seer of olive oil. Put the two together in a vessel and heat on the water bath for 30 mins. Remove and place in the sun for a month. Finally strain.

PUMELO OIL

Procedure: Peel off the green skin of pumelos and mince them with a knife. Take half and put in a vessel. Pour into it one seer good olive oil. Then heat the vessel on the water bath for half an hour. Remove and cover up the mouth of the vessel closely. Place it in the sun every day for one month. Then strain and bottle. The oil will be nicely scented.

ROSE OIL

The rose oil of India or as it is more popularly known, the otto of rose, was known all over the world in olden days and had the reputation of being the finest quality. Even to-day the small quantity of rose oil that is produced in India is as good as, if not superior to the Bulgarian rose oil. It is of vital importance to the country that the manufacture of rose oil in India should be undertaken on a much larger scale than hitherto. Ghazipur, which was once known all the world over as the centre of Indian rose oil, now produces roses on a very small scale on account of degradation of the species and the impoverishment of the soil and the centre of gravity for the production of rose oil has shifted to Barwana in Aligarh District of U.P. The season for roses in Barwana lasts for only six weeks, from the middle of March till the end of April, and it is reported that during this period as much as 200 maunds of rose petals are distilled per day and at the height of the season, which lasts for only about a week, the arrivals of flowers come to as much as 1,000 maunds per day. Most of the rose petals are, however, used up for the manufacture of rose attar and only about 5 to 7 lbs. of pure otto of rose is produced per annum. The distillation at Barwana is carried out by distillers from Kanauj by old methods and it is reported that about 13,000 lbs. of rose petals give about 1 lb. of rose oil, which means an yield of about .001 per cent; if a more modern method of distillation is adopted, it should be possible to obtain a higher yield. Systematic study of the manufacture of otto of rose by modern methods has been carried out by the Industries Department of the United Provinces and they have stated that the yield of oil can be raised to as much as 0.15 per cent by using an improved type of still, i.e., we can obtain from the existing crop of flowers at Barwana ten times more oil than what the crude method of distillation yields.

SANDALWOOD OIL

Sandalwood oil is obtained from the wood of the sandal trees which grow largely in the forests of Mysore, Coorg and Bombay Presidency. The wood is commercially valued according to size, weight, physical appearance, etc., and has varied domestic uses. The wood is rich in oil and according to the research carried out at the Forest Research Institute, Dehra Dun, the oil is found in both billets and roots. The wood is generally disintegrated into small fine powder before it is taken to the still for the extraction of the oil. The manufacture of sandalwood oil is conducted chiefly in Mysore and on a moderate scale at Kuppam, Mettur, Bombay, Kanauj and Karkal (S.K.) Most of the sandalwood oil factories operate modern stills with steam and the quality of the Indian oil is approved all over the world. There are, however, some factories in Mangalore which still extract the oil by crude methods of distillation, but their production is negligible and they are thus of no importance. With the development of the soap, toilet and perfumery industry and larger manufacture of pharmaceutical goods in India, there is every reason to believe that the manufacture of sandalwood oil will progress still further in the years to come.

Procedure: Take 5 srs. of sandalwood dust and 10 srs. of water. Put the two together in a suitable earthenware vessel for 48 hours. Then place on the water bath at steam heat for half an hour. Remove the vessel, cover it with a fine piece of cloth and place it in the hot sun. After a time a thin film will form on the surface of the decoction. Pick it out gently with a feather or cotton swab and put it gently in a clean phial. A similar layer will appear again and again on the freshly exposed surface. Pick out the films as soon, and as many times, as they are formed. Close the mouth of the phial air-tight, place in the sun for a month and store it away.

SALRESIN OR CHUA OIL

The oil is extracted by crude methods in Cuttack from Sal resion (Shorea Robusta) which is an exudation from sal trees which grow in Orissa. A systematic investigation of this oil would be desirable as it is reported that some years ago, as much as 1,000 lbs. of oil was extracted every day and was consumed by Kanauj distillers in the manufacture of incenses and attars.

TURPENTINE OIL

The oil of turpentine is obtained by steam distillation of oleo resin which exude from various pine trees which are tapped at regular intervals by incision. Three factories, one at Jallo in the Punjab and another at Bareilly in U.P. and a third in Kashmir are carrying out the manufacture of turpentine oil. Though turpentine oil as such has no use in the perfumery industry it is an important oil of commerce for paint and varnish industries, as also in the manufacture of wax polish. Turpentine oil is also the starting material for the manufacture of terpineol (synthetic lilac), the economic manufacture of which, however, depends on the pinene contents, particularly the Alpha variety, of the oil. The turpentine oil produced in India is unfortunately poor in alpha pinene, the percentage of which is only about 30.

SECTION THREE
ESSENCES AND OTTOS

CHAPTER VIII
PREPARATION OF ESSENCES

Perhaps the most democratic form of luxury indulged in by all lovers of perfumery is the essence, which is in principle an alcoholic solution dissolving essential oils either alone or in harmonious combination with others. The essence is also produced by distillation or by digestion. The pleasant aroma of the essences and their cheapness render them a most popular form of handkerchief and general perfumes.

The manufacture of essences is comparatively an easy task and does not involve complicated processes. Only what is required of the manufacturer is clean and careful manipulation. The object in view should be to arrive at a preparation the odour of which is pleasant and persists for a pretty long time and which does not leave any residue on evaporation.

MODE OF PREPARATION

To attain this end, most scrupulous attention should be attached to the selection of the constituents which enter into the composition of essences. The principal of these are alcohol and the essential oils. The alcohol used should be of the best quality available and rectified, if possible. Crude alcohol invariably contains a lot of impurities and its use as basis spoils the whole preparation. For deodorisation of alcohol *See pages 20-21*.

The range of essential oils at the command of the essence manufacturers, thanks to the evolution of synthetic perfumes, is extensively large. The distinctly predominant odours the manufacturers are capable of producing are thus no doubt numerous but this also renders the task of selection of the perfumes and their combination all the more difficult. But in all cases fresh and the best quality oils should be employed, otherwise the preparation cannot be expected to be of a high order of excellence.

FLORAL EXTRACTS

The essential oils can often be replaced by the odoriferous bodies yielding the perfumes themselves. The raw odoriferous bodies are infused in rectified spirit. On prolonged maceration, the period depending upon the nature of the body and the easiness with which it yields up its perfumes, the essences are obtained. These essences generally go by the name of natural essences. But their manufacture is rather restricted and the majority of essences met with in the market is derived from artificial sources and are made from the essential oils. Of course the concentrated forms of natural essences can be preserved and may be diluted with spirit either alone or in combination with ohters to give the most delicate preparations.

CLASSES OF ESSENCES

It will be thus noticed that the essences may be broadly divided into two groups, natural and artificial. The latter allows of further division, viz., *Simple* and *Compound*. The simple essences which are generally of the cheapest type and of inferior quality are prepared by dissolving a single essential oil, or generally a cheap synthetic preparation, in a not too pure form of alcohol. The compound essences on the other hand—and the same remark holds good in the case of the handkerchief essences—entail the use of more than one essential oil; besides, these preparations are designed to conform strictly to the ideal types of essences, and hence require the use of the best quality alcohol and perfumes.

BLENDING

In preparing artificial essences too much attention cannot be devoted to blending of the perfumes which should be made in a judicious manner so that the combination gives out a most pleasant smell and appeals to the general taste. Harmony of blending is the biggest thing to be attained in the preparation of essences and when this is achieved, success is more than

Blending of the perfumes should be universally followed by keeping the whole for a certain time undisturbed for maturing. This allows the odour of the alcohol and the foreign odours in essential oils employed to disappear and conserve the resulting scent.

FILTERING AND PACKING

The preparation should always be filtered before final packing. Turbid and unclean preparations do not command respect. The solutions should be perfectly clear and transparent. Ordinarily it will be found that the filtered solutions often cause deposits to form at the bottom of the container on long standing. Hence the essences as a general rule are allowed to stand for a few weeks and then filtered so that no residue can form later on.

The packing of the essential oils in phials also demands expert knowledge. The vessels should be carefully washed and dried before the essence is poured into them. By no means the essence should be packed in wet or even moist phials; for the least trace of moisture is sufficient to upset the equilibrium of the product, to precipitate a part of the perfume essence and to modify the odour. The vessels should also be filled completely and no space should be left above the liquid; for, in such cases alcohol and essential oils being volatile substances may volatilise partially and thus cause deterioration of the preparation. The vessels should then be stored in cool and dark places. It has been found that under these conditions the essence gains in quality and sweetness and improves.

While putting in the market the essences should be packed in decent glass containers fitted with glass stoppers. By no means ordinary cork should be used as this is liable to be injured by the spirit contained within. Finally the phial is capsuled, finely labelled and packed in cardboard boxes either singly or three or six at a time.

CHAPTER IX

NATURAL ESSENCES

The chief application of floral extracts lies in the manufacture of handkerchief perfumes, scents, essences, etc. The process of preparation is essentially the same in every case. Freshly blooming scented flowers are selected, freed from green stalks and cleaned from dirt and dust. The picked flowers are then digested in spirit. When flowers are not available, essential oils of the flowers or substitutes may be employed. Where the spirit has not been defined, rectified spirit is to be understood. By proof spirit is meant a mixture of equal bulks of alcohol and water while spirit of wine stands for the alcohol of commerce. After a time the liquid is filtered and the scent carefully bottled.

BAKUL

Procedure: Take *Bakul* flowers 8 oz., clean and free from dust; put them in a stoppered phial and pour in 20 oz. Cologne spirit. Close the mouth. Leave aside for 3 days and filter. Again soak 12 oz. fresh flowers in the filtered spirit and leave aside undisturbed for 48 hours. Finally filter and put in a stoppered phial.

HENNA

Procedure: *Mehndi* flowers 8 oz., proof spirit 16 oz. Put these two ingredients together in a stoppered phial for 15 days. Wring out the flowers and throw them away. Put 12 oz. fresh flowers in this spirit and filter after 7 days. Store in a stoppered bottle.

MUSK HENNA

Procedure: Take 1/16 tollah pure musk; 10 oz. *Mehndi* flowers; 20 oz. spirit. First macerate the musk in the spirit and put it in a stoppered phial. Throw in the flowers; shake well; close up the mouth and set aside for 10 days. Filter and store in a stoppered phial.

KETAKI

Procedure: Procure 6 oz. pollens of *Ketaki* flowers and 6 oz. tender leaves of the same plant, also 24 oz. proof spirit. Finally chop the leaves. Put all these ingredients into a wide-mouthed stoppered phial for 20 days. Filter through filter paper.

BELA

Procedure: Take 16 oz. *Bela* flowers free from stalks and 20 oz. Cologne spirit. Put these two ingredients in a wide-mouthed stoppered phial for 48 hours. Wring out the flowers and put in 8 oz. fresh flowers. Set aside for 24 hours and then filter through filter paper. Store carefully in a stoppered phial.

MALLIKA

Procedure: Put together 8 oz. *Mallika* flowers free from stalks and 12 oz. proof spirit into a wide-mouthed stoppered phial. Wring out the flowers after 3 days and throw in 8 oz. fresh flowers. Leave aside for 48 hours and then filter through filter paper and store in a stoppered phial.

GANDHARAJ

Procedure: Take 200 *Gandharaj* flowers free from stalks and 32 oz. spirit of wine. Put the two together into a stoppered phial for 3 days and then wring out the flowers. Put in 200 fresh flowers and leave for 48 hours. Wring out the flowers; put in a third lot of 100 flowers and set aside for 24 hours. Finally filter through filter paper.

HASU-NO-HENNA

Procedure: Put together 16 oz. *Hasu-no-henna* flowers and 16 oz. spirit in a wide-mouthed stoppered phial for 24 hours. Filter through filter paper; throw away the exhausted flowers. Put in 16 oz. fresh flowers in the same spirit and leave aside for 24 hours. Repeat this process for 6 times; filter through a filter paper and finally put in a stoppered phial.

CHAMPAKA

Procedure: Procure 100 *Champaka* flowers and then put in a stoppered phial. Pour 24 oz. spirit of wine into it and leave for 48 hours. Strain the liquid and throw away the exhausted flowers.

Put in 200 fresh flowers and leave for 24 hours. Finally filter through filter paper and bottle.

JAHURI CHAMPAKA

Procedure: Take 100 *Jahuri Champaka* flowers and 20 oz. proof spirit. Put the two together into a wide-mouthed stoppered phial for 24 hours. Wring out the flowers, then throw in 100 fresh flowers and set aside for 24 hours. Repeat this for seven times. Finally filter through filter paper and store in a stoppered phial.

KANTALI CHAMPAKA

Procedure: Procure 250 *Kantali Champaka* flowers and spirit 20 oz. Put the two together into a wide-mouthed stoppered phial, and close the mouth tightly. Strain after 15 days and throw away the exhausted flowers. Soak a fresh batch of 250 flowers into the spirit and filter after 48 hours. Store in a stoppered phial.

ROSE

Procedure: Procure 16 oz. dried buds of Rose (any scented variety) and 20 oz. spirit of wine. Put the two together into a wide-mouthed stoppered phial for 20 days. Filter through filter paper and store in a stoppered phial.

TUBEROSE

Procedure: Put 8 oz. *Tuberose* and 12 oz. proof spirit together into a wide-mouthed phial for 7 days. Strain and throw away the exhausted flowers. Put 8 oz. fresh flowers into the spirit; close up the mouth and set aside for 15 days. Put in a stoppered phial.

CHAMELI

Procedure: Take 12 oz. *Chameli* flowers free from stalks, put in a wide-mouthed stoppered phial and pour in 16 oz. Cologne spirit. Leave for 48 hours, strain and throw away the flowers. Put in 8 oz. fresh flowers, leave for 24 hours, then filter and store in a stoppered phial.

JASMINE

Procedure: Procure 16 oz. single *Jasmine* free from stalks and 12 oz. spirit. Put these two together into a wide-mouthed stoppered phial for 24 hours. Strain and throw away the exhausted flowers. Put in 8 oz. fresh flowers, close up the mouth tightly and leave for 24 hours. Finally filter through filter paper and store in a stoppered phial.

KHUS

Procedure: Procure 12 oz. *Khus* root; pick them and free them from dirt. Pound them finely. Soak the roots in 16 oz. spirits of wine and put the two together into a wide-mouthed stoppered phial. After a month filter through filter paper and put in a stoppered phial.

JANTI

Procedure: - Procure 8 oz. *Janti* flowers free from stalks; put in wide-mouthed stoppered phial and pur in 12 oz. spirit. Strain after 48 hours and throw away the exhausted flowers. Put in a fresh lot of 12 oz. flowers and filter through filter paper after 24 hours. Finally store in a stoppered phial.

ORANGE

Procedure: Procure 8 oz. dried peels of Orange and mince them fine. Soak them in 12 oz. spirit in a wide-mouthed stoppered phial. Close up its mouth and set aside for 1 month. Finally filter through filter paper and store in a stoppered phial.

AMBERGRIS

Procedure: Put 12 dr. Ambergris in a stoppered bottle and pour into it 3 pints of Cologne spirit. Close the mouth tightly and set aside for a month. Finally filter and store in a stoppered phial.

MUSK

Procedure: Macerate thoroughly 24 grs. of pure Musk in a stone mortar. Dissolve the same in 16 oz. spirit of wine and put the solution in a stoppered phial for 20 days. Shake once a day for 10 minutes every time. Finally filter and store in a stoppered phial.

PATCHOULI

Procedure: Procure 12 oz. clean and dry leaves of *Patchouli* and 12 oz. proof spirit. Put these two together into wide-mouthed stoppered phial; close the mouth tightly and set aside for one month. Then filter through filter paper and store in a stoppered phial.

CLOVES

Procedure: Take 1 ch. picked and cleaned Cloves and 20 oz. spirit of wine. Put the two together into wide-mouthed stoppered phial for a month. Then filter and store in a stoppered phial.

LAVENDER

Procedure: Take fresh Lavender flowers 20 oz. and spirit 32 oz. Put the two together into a stoppered phial. Close the mouth and leave for 1 month. Filter through filter paper and store in a stoppered phial.

PUMELO

Procedure: Procure Pumelo flowers, free from stalks, 8 oz. and spirit of wine 16 oz. Put them in a wide-mouthed stoppered phial for 48 hours. Strain and wring out the flowers and put in 8 oz. of fresh flowers. Set aside for 48 hours and strain as before. Again add 8 oz. of fresh flowers and filter after 48 hours. Pack in stoppered phials.

CASSIA

Procedure: Take oil of Cassia 4 dr. and Cologne spirit 12 oz. Keep in a stoppered bottle for 15 days and shake the bottle daily for 5 minutes. Finally strain and pack.

WHITE ROSE

Procedure: 16 oz. petals of white rose are put in a wide-mouthed bottle; 16 oz. of spirit is poured over them and the mouth is then closed. After 3 days, strain and reject the exhausted flowers. Again introduce 8 oz. of fresh flowers and close the mouth. After 48 hours filter and pack.

ORANGE

Procedure: 2 drs. of oil Neroli are taken in a bottle. 20 oz. of spirit is poured over it and the mouth of the bottle is closed. After 15 days filter and add 1 dr. of oil Neroli. Keep in stoppered phials.

BERGAMOT

Procedure: Oil of Bergamot 4 oz. and spirit of wine 30 oz. are taken in a stoppered bottle and kept for 7 days. Finally filter and then pack.

VIOLET

Procedure: 8 oz. of finely powdered orris root is digested in 24 oz. of spirit of wine in a stoppered bottle. Set aside for 1 month. Finally filter and phial.

ROSE GERANIUM

Procedure: Put 4 dr. of oil of Rose Geranium and 16 oz. of spirit in a stoppered bottle and keep for 20 days. Then filter and phial.

LEMON

Procedure: 8 oz. of fresh lemon peels are minced and digested in 20 oz. of spirit of wine in a stoppered bottle. Mix well and set aside for three days in a warm place. Finally filter and phial.

SANDALWOOD

Procedure: Mix together 4 oz. of Sandalwood dust and 8 oz. of white chalk and digest in 12 oz. of spirit and set aside in a stoppered bottle for a week. Then strain through filter paper and to the filtrate add 1 oz. of sandal oil. Store in a bottle for 2 weeks before phialing.

Procedure: Finely powdered Sandalwood dust weighing 16 oz. is digested in 12 oz. of Cologne spirit in a wide-mouthed stoppered vessel. Set aside for a month, then filter and pack.

CHAPTER X

ARTIFICIAL ESSENCES

The preparation of simple essences consists primarily in mixing some Heiko perfume, such as heiko bela, heiko rose, heiko patchouli, heiko jasmine, heiko musk, heiko chameli, etc. in rectified spirit 60 over-proof.

The method of preparation is as easy as it is simple. The whole is allowed to mature for a fortnight or more, during which period the containing bottle is shaken three times daily for 15 minutes every time. The usual proportion recommended by perfumers is 1 oz. of the heiko scent in 48 oz. of the spirit. Sometimes a small quantity of musk, essence of musk or essence of ambergris is added to render the perfume more persistent and also to improve the odour. The perfumes may be packed in tubes.

SIMPLE ESSENCES

The few recipes given below offer the clue to the manufacture of many others of similar type:

1. Heiko Lily, 1 oz.; Essence Amber, 2 oz.; Spirit, 48 oz.

2. Heiko Tuberose, 1 oz.; Essence Ambergris, 1 oz.; Spirit, 48 oz.

3. Heiko Lily of the Valley, 4 dr.; Essence Musk, 1 oz.; Spirit, 24 oz.

4. Heiko White Rose, 4 dr.; Musk, 2 dr.; Spirit, 24 oz.

ESSENCES FROM COUNTRY OTTOS

Simple essences are also prepared by dissolving country made ottos in spirit with the addition of benzoic acid. The mode of preparation is exactly the same, only the time of maturing is lengthened to one month. A few typical recipes follow:

1. Otto of Jasmine or Santal, 1½ tollah; Spirit, 24 oz.; Benzoic Acid, 15 gr.

2. Otto of Henna or Bakul, 2 tollahs; Spirit 24 oz.; Benzoic Acid, 15 gr.

3. Oil of Chameli Flowers, 1 tollah; Benzoic Acid, 8 gr.; Musk 2 gr.; Spirit, 16 oz.

HANDKERCHIEF ESSENCES

The essences prepared according to the process described above may be mixed in suitable proportions to give cheap handkerchief essences as follows:

I

Essence	Rose	16 oz.
"	Keora	2 oz.
"	Jasmine	2 oz.
"	Lily of the Valley	3 oz.
"	Amber	1 oz.

Procedure: Mix together: Shake for 15 minutes, three times a day for three days. Then use.

II

Essence	Chameli	16 oz.
"	Rose	4 oz.
"	Jasmine	2 oz.
"	Neroli	1 oz.
"	Amber	$1/2$ oz.
"	Musk	$1/2$ oz.

Procedure: The same.

COMPOUND ESSENCES

The preparation of compound essences taxes the best skill of the perfumers. As already remarked much would depend upon perfect manipulations. For marketing, pack them in decent phials with glass stoppers. A few recipes follow:

FORGET-ME-NOT

Essence	Amber	2 dr.
"	Orange	1 dr.
"	Vanilla Bean	4 dr.
"	Ylang Ylang	4 dr.
"	Jasmine	3 dr.
"	Rose	8 dr.
"	Sandal	2 dr.
Otto	Neroli	1 dr.
"	Bergamot	2 dr.
"	Musk	30 minims.
Rectified Spirit		2 bottles

Procedure: Add the ingredients one by one in a big vessel and have them thoroughly mixed together with shaking. Put the whole air-tight in a stoppered vessel for a fortnight during which period shake it thrice daily for 15 minutes at a time. Finally filter through filter paper and phial. The aroma of this preparation is very delightful and lasting.

REMEMBER-ME

Otto	Jasmine	1 dr.
Flora	Jasmine	2 dr.
Otto	Orange Flower	1 dr.
"	Rose (Turkish)	30 minims.
Oil	Cloves	15 minims.
"	Geranium Rose	4 dr.
"	Citron	3 dr.
"	Bergamot	2 dr.
Oil Lavender (English)		1 dr.
Essence	Amber	2 oz.
"	Musk	1 oz.
Rectified Spirit		2 bottles

Procedure: As in Forget-me-not.

SIR WALTER SCOTT

Extract	Rose or Istambal	1	dr.
Otto	Orange Flower	30	minims.
”	Bergamot	30	minims.
”	Lavender	15	minims.
Essence Jasmine		1	oz.
”	Musk	1	oz.
Alcohol		1	bottle

Procedure: As in Forget-me-not.

ESSENCE JASMINE

Otto of Jasmine	1	dr.
Flora Jasmine	2	dr.
Heiko Jasmine	1	dr.
Otto de Rose	30	minims.
Essence Neroli	2	dr.
” Musk	2	oz.
Alcohol	1	bottle

Procedure: As in Forget-me-not.

GLORI DAUCHER

Essence Victoria	12	oz.
Extract Rose or Istambal	1	dr.
Otto Sandal	30	minims.
” Jasmine	1	dr.
” de Rose (Virgin)	1	dr.
Heiko Amber	2	dr.
” Pitunia	1	dr.
” Tuberose	30	minims.
Rectified Spirit	2	bottles

Procedure: Mix the ingredients one by one with shaking. Put the whole air-tight into a stoppered vessel and shake it thrice daily for 15 minutes at a time for not less than a month. Finally filter and pack in phials.

KISS-ME-QUICK

Essence	Jasmine	2 oz.
"	Orange Flower	2 oz.
Spirit	Tonka Bean	½ oz.
"	Ambergris	1 dr.
Cologne	Spirit	12 oz.

Procedure: As in Glori Daucher.

JOCKEY CLUB

Essence of Rose		4 oz.
"	Cassia	2 oz.
"	Jasmine	4 oz.
"	Ambergris	4 dr.
Tincture Orris		4 dr.

Procedure: As in Glori Daucher.

MUSK ROSE

Otto de Rose		1 dr.
Sandal Oil		1 dr.
Musk		2 dr.
Essence	Vanilla	1 oz.
"	Jasmine	1 oz.
Benzoic Acid		15 gr.
Spirit		1 bottle

Procedure: As in Glori Daucher.

ESSENCE VICTORIA

Otto de Rose (Virgin)		2 dr.
Oil	Neroli	2 dr.
Otto of	Coriander	16 minims.
Oil of	Bergamot	4 dr.
"	Pimento	24 minims.
"	Lavender	16 minims.
Musk		4 gr.
Benzoic Acid		2 dr.
Spirit		4 bottles

Procedure: As in Glori Daucher.

AMERICAN BEAUTY

Otto de Rose (Virgin)	4 dr.
Essence Neroli	1 oz.
Heiko Rose	2 dr.
Essence Jasmine	1 oz.
Otto Cedar Wood	12 minims.
Musk	8 gr.
Benzoic Acid	1 dr.
Alcohol	4 bottles.

Procedure: As in Glori Daucher.

ESSENCE TUBEROSE LILY

Heiko Lily	4 dr.
" Jasmine	1 dr.
" Tuberose	2 dr.
Otto de Rose	30 minims.
Oil Bergamot	1 dr.
Essence Amber	1 dr.
Alcohol	1 bottle

Procedure: The constituents are mixed together thoroughly one by one and the whole is then allowed to stand undisturbed for 7 days. Then filter, and shake the whole for 15 minutes at a time, thrice daily for 7 days. Finally pack in phials.

ESSENCE ROSE

Extract Rose or Istambal	2 dr.
Magnesium Carbonate	4 "
Alcohol	1 bottle

Procedure: First incorporate well the extract rose with the magnesium carbonate in a stone mortar and then add to it the alcohol. Shake the whole thrice daily, 15 minutes at a time, for a fortnight and then filter and phial. The residue left after filtering in the blotting paper when dissolved in one bottle of distilled water will give rise to a very good quality of rose water.

NIZAM MONTE CRISTO

Rectified	Spirit	24	oz.
Extract	Rose or Istambal	30	minims.
Otto de	Rose (Virgin)	30	minims.
Heiko	White Rose	1	dr.
Otto	Keora	15	minims.
"	Orange Flower	10	minims.
Essence	Chameli	1	oz.
"	Jasmine	1	oz.
"	Tuberose	1	oz.
"	Ambergris	1	oz.

Procedure: Into the rectified spirit add the ingredients one by one and shake well for 5 minutes after each such addition. Finally keep the whole in a stoppered bottle and shake thrice daily, 10 minutes at a time, for seven days together. Finally filter and phial. The preparation is quite a novel invention.

SULTANA

Spirit		2	bottles.
Otto de	Rose (Turkish)	1	dr.
Tincture	Orris Root	4	oz.
"	Musk	2	oz.
Essence	Sandal	1	oz.
"	Bergamot	2	oz.
"	Lilac	4	oz.
"	Lavender	4	oz.
Flora	Jasmine	1	dr.
Otto	Keora	4	dr.

Procedure: As in Nizam Monte Cristo.

LAVENIA

Spirit		24	oz.
Oil of	Lavender (Mitchams)	50	minims.
"	Orange	30	minims.
"	Neroli	30	minims.
"	Rosemary	1	dr.
"	Bergamot	1	dr.

Otto de	Rose	15	minims.
"	Keora	1	dr.
Essence	Amber	2	oz.
"	Cedrat	4	dr.
"	Narcissus	4	dr.
"	Jasmine	4	dr.

Procedure: As in Nizam Monte Cristo.

JUNG BAHADUR

Spirit		2	bottles
Heiko	Jasmine	4	dr.
Flora	Jasmine	4	dr.
Otto	Chameli	2	dr.
"	Keora	1	dr.
"	Sandal	1	dr.
"	Orange Flower	1	dr.
"	Rose (Turkish)	1	dr.
Essence	Civet	2	oz.
"	Amber	1	oz.
"	Heliotrope	4	oz.
"	Rose Geranium	4	oz.

Procedure: As in Nizam Monte Cristo.

JUBILEE RAJANIGANDHA

Spirit		100	oz.
Heiko	Tuberose	2	oz.
Heiko	Pitunia	2	dr.
"	Hyacynth	1	dr.
"	Oppoponex	1	dr.
Flora	Jasmine	1	oz.
"	Narcissus	30	minims.
Oil	Neroli	1	dr.
"	Bergamot	1	dr.
"	Lavender (English)	2	dr.
"	Sandal	1	dr.
Otto de	Rose (Virgin)	1	dr.

Procedure: As in Nizam Monte Cristo. The preparation is most pleasing.

MADHUMALATI

Essence	Lilac	6 oz.
,,	Cananga	6 oz.
,,	Rose Geranium	8 oz.
,,	Vanilla	2 oz.
,,	Ambergris	2 oz.
,,	Bergamot	4 oz.
,,	Lavender	6 oz.
,,	Sandal	3 oz.
Oil	Neroli	1 dr.
Otto de	Rose	1 dr.

Procedure: The ingredients are put one by one in a bottle, the mouth of which is then closed. Shake the bottle thrice daily, 10 minutes at a time, for fifteen days when the preparation will be ready for use.

CANANGA KUSUM

Spirit		1 bottle
Otto	Orange Flower	1 dr.
,,	de Rose	30 minims.
,,	Keora	1 dr.
Oil de	Rose Geranium	2 dr.
,,	Lavender (English)	1 dr.
Essence	Sandal	1 oz.
,,	Citron	1 oz.
,,	Cassia	$1/2$ oz.
,,	Amber	2 oz.

Procedure: Into the spirit contained in the bottle add the essential oils one by one, shake the bottle for 3 minutes each time. The bottle is then closed airtight and kept in a cool place for 15 days. Shake the bottle twice daily for 10 minutes every day for a fortnight. Finally filter the whole and phial in a stoppered vessel.

MARSENIL

Alcohol		24	oz.
Extract	Rose or Istambal	1	dr.
Heiko	Rose	30	minims.
Otto	de Rose	30	minims.
"	Jasmine (or Heiko)	1	dr.
Flora	Jasmine	30	minims.
Heiko	Amber	1	dr.
"	Lily	1	dr.
Oil	Rose Geranium	1	dr.
Essence	Musk	1	oz.
"	Keora	1	oz.

Procedure: Take the alcohol in a big bottle and add the other ingredients one by one. The bottle should be shaken for 5 minutes after the addition of each of the ingredients. When all the ingredients are added into the alcohol, the bottle is stoppered air-tight and kept in that position for a fortnight. The bottle should, however, be shaken thrice daily, 10 minutes at a time. Finally the whole is filtered and phialed. The preparation is exquisite and the scent lasts for 7 days.

LILY BLOSSOM

Spirit		48	oz.
Heiko	Lily of the Valley (New)	4	dr.
Heiko	Lily	2	dr.
"	Lime Blossom	2	dr.
Flora	Jasmine (or Heiko)	1	dr.
Otto	de Rose	30	minims.
"	Khus	1	dr.
Oil	Neroli	1	dr.
"	Sandal	1	dr.
Essence	Amber	1	oz.
"	Civet	1	oz.
"	Musk	½	oz.

Procedure: As in Marsenil.

CHANDRA MALLIKA

Alcohol		1	bottle
Heiko	Hyacynth	1	bottle
Heiko	Lily	1	dr
"	Amber	1	dr.
"	Oppoponax	1	dr.
Otto	Keora	1	dr.
Heiko	Reseda	1	dr.
"	Pitunia	1	dr.

Procedure: As in Marsenil.

CHERRY LAUREL

Spirit		24	oz.
Oil	Cherry Laurel	4	dr.
Heiko	Amber	1	dr.
Otto	de Rose	15	minims.
"	Keora	1	dr.
Essence	Jasmine	1	oz.
"	Musk	1	oz.
"	Neroli	1	oz.
"	Bergamot	1	oz.

Procedure: Add into the spirit the other ingredients one by one, shaking the whole for 5 minutes after each such addition. Then keep the whole in a stoppered bottle for 10 days and shake it thrice daily for 5 minutes at a time during the period. Finally filter and phial.

EMPEROR

Spirit		48	oz.
Essence	Neroli	2	dr.
"	Amber	2	oz.
"	Musk	1	oz.
"	Violet	4	oz.
Oil	Lavender (English)	1	dr.
"	Primento	30	minims.

Oil	Coriander	30	minims.
Essence	Bergamot	4	oz.
"	Neroli	4	oz.
"	Jasmine	8	oz.
"	White Rose	6	oz.
Otto de Rose		1	dr.

Procedure: As in Cherry Laurel.

CASHMERE BAKUL

Spirit		48	oz.
Otto	Bakul (Country)	3	dr.
Flora	Narcissus	4	dr.
Heiko	Narcissus	2	dr.
"	Pitunia	2	dr.
"	Amber	1	dr.
Essence	Mimosa	1	oz.
"	White Rose	1	oz.
"	Jasmine	4	oz.
"	Sandal	1	oz.
"	Neroli	1	oz.

Procedure: As in Cherry Laurel.

CORONATION

Alcohol		48	oz.
Otto	Nageswar	4	dr.
"	Chameli	1	dr.
"	Bela	1	dr.
"	Henna	1	dr.
"	Keora	2	dr.
Flora	Jasmine	1	dr.
Oil	Neroli	30	minims.
"	Bergamot	30	minims.
"	Sandal	40	minims.
"	Lavender	1	dr.
Otto de Rose		30	minims.

| Heiko | Lily of the Valley (New) | 1 dr. |
| " | Amber | 2 dr. |

Procedure: As in Cherry Laurel.

CHERRY VANILLA

Spirit		24 oz.
Heiko	Millefluers	2 oz.
"	Opela	1 dr.
Tincture	Vanilla	4 oz.
Oil	Cherry Laurel	1 dr.
Otto	Orange Flower	30 minims.
"	Rose Geranium (French)	4 dr.
Essence	Ambergris	1 oz.
"	Bergamot	2 oz.
Otto de Rose		30 minims.

Procedure: As in Cherry Laurel.

PRINCE ROSE

Spirit		36 oz.
Pure	Musk	12 gr.
Extract	Rose or Istambal	90 gr.
Otto de	Rose	1 dr.
"	Jasmine	1 dr.
"	Orange Flower	30 minims.
Essence	Violet	4 oz.
"	Amber	4 oz.
Essence	Vanilla	1 oz.

Procedure : - As in Cherry Laurel.

BOUQET EMPRESS

Spirit		48 oz.
Oil of	Rose Geranium	4 dr.
"	Geranium	2 dr.
"	Neroli	1 dr.
"	Lemon	30 minims.

Oil of	Bergamot	30	minims.
"	Sassafras	4	dr.
"	Lavender (Mitchams)	1	dr.
Heiko	Jasmine	30	minims.
"	Lily	2	dr.
"	Amber	2	dr.
"	Musk	1	dr.
Essence Vanilla		3	dr.
Oil	Hasu-no-Hena	4	dr.

Procedure: As in Cherry Laurel.

DURBAR

Spirit	Cassia	4	oz.
"	Violet	8	oz.
Oil	Bergamot	4	dr.
"	Citron	1	oz.
Flora	Jasmine	4	dr.
Otto	Orange Flower	1	dr.
" de Rose		30	minims.
Essence Amber		4	oz.
"	Rose Geranium	6	oz.
"	Lily of the Valley	8	oz.
"	Sandal	1	oz.
Oil	Lavender	30	minims.
Tincture Grass		to colour.	

Procedure: The ingredients are mixed with shaking one by one. Keep aside in a stoppered vessel for three days and during that period shake the vessel thrice daily for 5 minutes at a time. Finally filter and pack.

VICEROY VERBENA

Spirit		72	oz.
Heiko	Verbena	1	oz.
Essence	Amber	3	oz.
"	Musk	1	oz.

Tincture	Orris	2 oz.
Oil	Neroli	30 minims.
Otto de	Rose	1 dr.
"	Sandal	1 dr.
Flora	Jasmine	2 dr.
Oil	Lavender (Mitchams)	1 dr.

Procedure: As in Durbar.

NAPOLEON LILY

Spirit		24 oz.
Heiko	Lily	4 oz.
Essence	Amber	1 oz.
"	Tuberose	½ oz.
"	New-mown hay	½ oz.
Otto de	Rose	30 minims.
Heiko	Jasmine	1 dr.
"	Khus (or Otto)	30 minims.
Otto	Sandal	30 minims.
"	Keora	30 minims.

Procedure: As in Durbar.

CHYPRE

Oil of	Rosemary	100 minims.
"	Bitter Orange	½ oz.
"	Petit Grain	2 dr.
"	Bergamot	2½ dr.
"	Neroli	45 minims.
"	Alcohal	80 oz.

Procedure: Mix and after 4 days add 10 oz. of distilled water. Allow to stand for a fortnight and filter.

HELIOTROPE

Heliotropin	160 grains
Vanillin	24 grains
Coumarin	16 grains

Essence of Musk	160	minims.
Ylang Ylang Oil (Syn.)	60	minims.
Geraniol	32	minims.
Benzaldehyde	8	minims.
Rectified Spirit	1	gallon

ESSENCE BOUQUET

Oil of	Neroli	15	minims.
"	Lemon	1	dr.
"	Bergamot	1/2	dr.
Cassie	Extract	1	oz.
Essence of Ambergris		1	oz.
Tincture of Orris		1	oz.
Spirit of Rose		8	oz.
Alcohol		5	oz.

LILAC

Terpineol	2	fl. oz.
Vanillin	40	grains
Jasmine Otto (Syn.)	2	fl. dr
Geraniol	32	minims.
Palmarosa Oil	32	minims.
Bergamot Oil	60	minims.
Rectified Spirit	1	gallon

HYACINTH

Hyacinthin	1	dr.
Oil of Neroli	10	drops
Essence of Musk	50	drops
Tincture Benzoin	10	drops
Jasmine Extract	10	dr.
Orange Flower Water	5	dr.
Alcohol to make	10	oz.

BRIDAL BOUQUET

Oil of Sandal	½	dr.
Rose Extract	4	oz.

Jasmine Extract	4	oz.
Orange Flower Extract	16	oz.
Essence of Vanilla	1	oz.
Essence of Musk	2	oz.
Tincture of Storax	2	oz.

ORIENTAL BOUQUET

I

Oil of Lavender	100	drops
Otto of Rose	1	dr.
Jasmine Extract	2½	oz.
Essence of Vanilla	2½	oz.
Alcohol to produce	40	oz.

II

Heliotropin	15	grains
Coumarin	8	grains
Oil of Neroli	2	dr.
" Geranium	2½	dr.
Essential Oil of Almond	5	drops
Jasmine Extract	10	oz.
Alcohol	30	oz.

III

Heliotropin	60	grams
Terpineol	50	grams
Bergamot oil	30	grams
Phenyl acetaldehyde	24	grams
Syn. Musk	5	grams
Cananga Oil	5	grams
Alcohol	10	litres

IV

Terpineol	15	parts
Vanillin	1	part
Musk Ambrette	1	part
Ylang Oil	1	part

Benzyl Acetate	2 parts
Linalol	1 part
Ionone	1 part
Cananga Oil	1 part
Infusion Ambrette Seeds, 20 per cent.	25 parts
Alcohol	1000 parts

CHAPTER XI

PREPARATION OF OTTOS

There is an air of freshness associated with the natural floral ottos rarely discernible even in the best of artificial essences. Moreover, the scent of the former is of more permanent nature and not at all evanescent, like the latter. It is, therefore, quite natural that floral ottos find wide application in the indigenous art of perfumery in preference to others.

The reputation of Indian attars once spread beyond the boundaries of India. Place like Ghazipur, Jaunpur and Kanauj, the important centres of production, were well-known throughout the world. Unfortunately the attar industry to-day is in a deplorable condition. The decline may be attributed to development of wide range of synthetic perfumes in the West which are now being used in the production of toilet goods, soap, confectionery, etc., etc.

Ottos may be described as blends of flower oils with sandalwood oil in varying proportions. The quality of the otto is in fact determined by the proportion of floral oil used in its preparation.

FLORAL OTTOS

The fundamental principle underlying the preparation of floral ottos is similar in every case while the basis of all of them is the same. Freshly bloomed flowers before their full expansion are selected as they are the most fragrant. They are stalked, removing the green calyxes and gently freed from dirt and dust without injuring the petals. Care should be exercised in this respect, otherwise the otto will be contaminated. They are steeped in water or sandal oil, heated on the water bath or warmed by the sun and finally filtered through a funnel. The filtered otto is collected in a stoppered phial and placed in the sun for a number of days to clarify. A sediment is allowed to form at the bottom so that the supernatant liquid gradually gets thin, limpid and clear.

ROSE

I

Procedure: Procure 4 oz. fresh rose petals all of one colour (say, crimson) and free them from dust, etc. Next take 16 oz. sandal oil in another vessel and heat on the water bath for half an hour. Take away, throw the petals into the oil, cover up and set aside for one hour. Then squeeze out the oil from from the soaked petals and heat the oil again on the water bath for half an hour. Take away and soak in it 4 oz. fresh petals for an hour. Squeeze out the oil, and repeat the above process once again. Finally squeeze out the oil and store in a stoppered phial. Put in the sun for one month and it will be clear.

II

Procedure: Procure rose petals of one colour and lay out ½ inch thick in a vessel. Cover them with a clean piece of rag moistened with sandal oil and folded 4 times. The cloth should be thoroughly wetted by rasping. Lay out over the rag another lot of rose petals. Make up in this way sixteen layers. Then close up the mouth of the vessel and place in the sun for 15 days. Finally press out the otto. Store in a stoppered phial and place in the sun for a month to clarify.

III

Procedure: The cleaned petals are placed in a clean vessel of glass, porcelain or earthenware, and covered up with pure water (rain or spring). Now place this vessel in some open space for a week or so to be warmed by the sun. After 3 or 4 days an oily substance will float on the surface which will appear like a scum the next day. This is rose otto. These oily spots must be removed by sponging with a cotton swab and squeezed into a phial.

About two lakhs of roses are required to prepare 2 ½ tolas of pure rose otto. But the ottos sold in the market are generally adulterated with sandal oil. The roses must be all of the same variety, otherwise the quality of the product will suffer.

IV

Procedure: Take 8 ch. of petals of red roses of the same variety. After freeing them of dirt and dust put them into a wide-mouthed glass bottle. Put in 30 grains of benzoic acid and pour in 8 ch. of pure sandal oil. Stopper the bottle closely and place in the sun for three days. Then squeeze out the digested petals and throw in 8 ch. fresh rose petals. Stopper the bottle and place in the sun. Repeat the process six or seven times. A concentrated otto of excellent quality will thus be obtained. Also see page ICI.

BELA

Procedure: Take 8 ch. freshly bloomed double or single *Bela* flowers (Arabian jasmine); white chalk, 2 ch.; sandal oil, 1 seer. First powder the chalk and boil it in water on an earthenware vessel. Remove after one hour, strain away the water and dry the chalk powder thoroughly. Now place the flowers on a wide-mouthed porcelain jar; throw in the chalk powder and cover up the jar. After 3 days throw out the withered flowers. The powder should be gently sifted and put in a glass vessel. Now pour in the sandal oil and put in the sun daily for a fortnight. Finally filter through a piece of flannel and the filtrate will be a good otto.

The bela otto is produced from jasmine flowers of Moghra variety which are grown at Kanauj, Jaunpur, Ghazipur and Sikandarpur. The Moghra flower is a variety of jasmine but is quite different to the pure jasmine. It may be stated that the crop of the former variety is 10 times as large as that of true jasmine. The bela otto has aroma quite different from that of jasmine. An "absolute" may be obtained from the flowers by the enfleurage process.

CHAMELI

Procedure: Take 2½ srs. stalked *Chameli* flowers Jasminum Grandiflorum. (Put into clean jar and strew) over them 15 grs. benzoic acid. Close up the mouth and set aside for 24 hours. Next day pour into it 24 oz. sandal oil, close up the mouth and place in the sun for 20 days. Then filter through filter paper on a funnel, store in a stoppered phial and place it in the dew for one month.

JASMINE

The jasmine otto is obtained from Jasminum Auriculatum Vahl known as *juhi*, which flowers in April and again in July to October.

Procedure: Petals of Jasmine, 2 ch.; sandal oil 8 ch. The stalks of the flowers must be gently removed with the help of a piece of broken glass avoiding contamination by hand. Then place ½ ch. of petals on a glass vessel, cover up with a piece of fine linen (muslin); pour on it 2 ch. of sandal oil. Then place another layer of ½ ch. of petals arranged in 4 similar layers. Close up the vessel and set aside for 24 hours. Then strain out the spent flowers, reject them and repeat the above process with fresh flowers, but with the same oil for half a dozen times. Press out the oil and store in a stoppered phial. Place in the sun for one month to clarify. A good otto will be obtained.

It may be further pointed out that in preparing the cheaper varieties of the otto, 6 to 8 maunds of flowers is added to about 10 lbs. of sandalwood oil whilst the superior quality is produced by storing the otto of one season for 3 or 4 years during which period fresh jasmine extract is added to it every year.

MALLIKA

Procedure: Procure a quantity of freshly bloomed flowers (Jasminum Angustifolium) and lay out a portion of it one inch thick in a spacious vessel. Spread over it some cleaned and beaten cotton, ½ inch thick, covering all sides. Lay out on it another layer of flowers and form in this way 10 layers. Pour on the top 1 sr. sandal oil, cover up the mouth of the vessel and place in the sun for 20 days. After that pour out its contents on to a piece of flannel and squeeze out the oil. Store it in a stoppered phial and place in the sun to clarify.

MADHUMALATI

Procedure: Take ½ sr. *Madhumalati* flowers. Gently free them from dust. Put them in an aluminium vessel. Pour 1 sr. sandal oil into them and heat on the water bath for 15 minutes. After 24 hours wring out the flowers. Steep in the oil another lot of ½ sr. flowers and heat on the water bath for 15 minutes.

Repeat the process 12 times. Finally strain through a piece of flannel. Put in a stoppered phial and place in the sun to clarify. Finally filter.

HENNA

Procedure: Put 4 oz. *Henna* flowers into a wide-mouthed bottle;

throw in 15 grs. benzoic acid and pour in 20 oz. clear sandal oil. Place in the sun for 16 days. Then filter through filter paper fitted in a funnel. Put the filtered oil again in the bottle and soak a fresh lot of 6 oz. flowers. Close the mouth and set aside for one month. Finally filter through filter paper and store in a stoppered phial.

MUSK HENNA

Procedure: Take 8 oz. *Mehndi* flowers; 6 grs. musk; and 12 oz. sandal oil. First macerate the musk with a little sandal oil in a stone mortar. Dilute it with the remainder of the oil and put in wide-mouthed bottle. Throw in the flowers, shake well, close up the mouth and set aside for one month. Finally filter through a funnel and store in a stoppered phial.

CHAMPAKA

Procedure: Put 500 freshly bloomed *Champaka* flowers in a jar and strew over them 15 grs. benzoic acid. Pour 24 oz. sandal oil into it, close up the mouth and place the phial in the sun and in the dew at night for one month. Finally filter through filter paper. Put in a stoppered phial and place in the sun for a fortnight to clarify.

KANTALI CHAMPAKA

Procedure: Procure 100 fresh and clean flowers and 1 sr. sandal oil. Put the two ingredients together in a vessel; close up the mouth and heat on the water bath for half an hour. Take away and leave aside for 24 hours. Strain through a funnel and separate the flowers. Put the oil in the above vessel and soak in it a fresh lot of 100 flowers. Heat on the water bath for half an hour and set aside for 24 hours. Separate the flowers as before and put the oil in the vessel. Soak in it a fresh lot of 100 flowers, cover the mouth and place in the sun for 16 days and in dew at night. After that filter through filter paper and store up in a stoppered phial. Place in the sun for one month to clarify and finally store in a stoppered phial.

JAHURI CHAMPAKA

Procedure: Procure 400 freshly bloomed *Jahuri Champaka* flowers, reject the green stalks and put in a porcelain jar. Strew over them 15 grs. benzoic acid and pour in 24 oz. sandal oil.

Place in the sun for 15 days, and squeeze out the otto. Put in a stoppered phial and place in the sun and in dew at night for one month.

DOLAN CHAMPAKA

Procedure: Procure 2,000 stalked *Dolan Champaka* flowers. Take 10 srs. of clear water in a large earthen bowl. Dissolve in it 2 dr. saltpetre and stir briskly. Now throw the flowers into it, mix gently and place in an open space. After seven days a thin film will appear on the surface. Remove this carefully with a feather without disturbing. Put in a stoppered phial. When all the films are collected, close the mouth and place in the sun for a month and in the dew at night.

NAGESWAR CHAMPAKA

Procedure: Procure 1 sr. selected and clean *Nageswar* flowers and 1 sr. sandal oil. Put the two ingredients together in a vessel, close up the mouth and heat on the water bath for half an hour. Take away, leave aside for 24 hours and press out the oil. Put the oil again into the vessel and soak in it 1 sr. picked flowers. Heat on the water bath for half an hour and then leave aside for 15 days in a cool place. Then press out the oil and store in a stoppered phial. Place in the sun and in dew at night for a month to clarify.

BAKUL

Procedure: Procure 5 srs. of picked *Bakul* flowers. Dirt and dust should be gently removed, otherwise the final product will be spoilt. Put the flowers in a glass, stone or earthenware vessel and fill up with 16 srs. of clean water. Dissolve 4 dr. salt in the water previously. Place the vessel in the sun continuously for 8 or 10 days in a place open to the sky. On the 4th or 5th day a thin oily film will appear on the surface; it will form into scum in a day or two. Carefully take this away with a feather or a cotton swab and put in a glass phial. Remove it as often as it forms. When all the scum is thus cleared, place the phial in the sun to clarify. Add 8 oz. sandal oil to 4 dr. extract.

GANDHARAJ

Procedure: Procure 5 srs. fresh *Gandharaj* flowers free from dirt and reject the stalks and green parts. Lay out ½ sr. of flowers at the bottom of a porcelain jar, strew over it 1 oz. magnesium carbonate. Spread out on it another layer of ½ sr. flowers at the bottom of a porcelain jar, strew over it 1 oz. magnesium carbonate. Spread out on it another layer of ½ sr. flowers and strew over it 1 oz. magnesium carbonate. In this way make up 10 layers. Close up the mouth of the vessel and place in the sun and in dew at night for a fortnight. Now separate the flowers after dripping and pour into the residue of the jar ½ sr. sandal oil. Place the vessel in the sun for 15 days and finally filter through filter paper. Place in the sun for a month to clarify.

HASU-NO-HENNA

Procedure: Pick bunches of *Hasu-no-henna* flowers just at dusk weighing 5 srs. Lay out 1 sr. at the bottom of a vessel and spread over it a piece of clean rag covering all sides. Lay out on it another layer of 1 sr. flowers and form in this way 5 layers with rags intervening. Finally cover up with rag and pour 20 oz. pure sandal oil. Cover up the mouth and place in the sun for 20 days. Press out the oil and store in a stoppered phial. Place in the sun for a month to clarify.

PATCHOULI

Procedure: Take 2½ srs. of *Patchouli* leaves; pick, dust and clean, and pound them into fine powder. Then lay out ½ sr. of the powder at the bottom of a vessel and spread on it a piece of cotton cloth. Lay out on it another layer of ½ sr. powder. In this way form 5 layers covering the last one with cotton cloth. Pour on the top 1 sr. sandal oil, close up the mouth of the vessel and place in the sun for a month and in dew at night. After that press out the oil and store in a stoppered phial. Finally place in the sun for 1 month to clarify.

TUBEROSE

Procedure: Take 1 sr. fresh *Tuberose*, put them in a vessel together with 1 sr. sandal oil, close up the mouth and heat on the water bath for 20 minutes. Leave aside for 12 hours. Then squeeze out the oil and put the oil again into the vessel. Soak a fresh lot of 1 sr. flowers and repeat the process for seven times. Finally press out the oil and store up in a stoppered phial. Place in the sun for a month and in dew at night to clarify.

KEORA

Procedure: Take half seer pollen of *Keora*, one seer tender leaves of the plant finely minced and 1 sr. good sandal oil. Put these three ingredients mixed together in a porcelain jar and close up the mouth tightly. Place in the sun for a month and then press out the oil. Store in a stoppered phial and place in the sun for a month to clarify.

KAMINI

Procedure: Take 1 sr. *Kamini* flowers free from stalk, put in an aluminium vessel, pour into it 1 sr. sandal oil, close up the mouth and heat on the water bath for half an hour. Set aside for 24 hours and then sequeeze out the otto. Put it again into the vessel and soak in it a fresh lot of ½ sr. flowers, and repeat the process twice. Finally press out the oil and store in a stoppered phial.

KHUS

Procedure: Procure 10 srs. of *Khus* root; free them from dirt and cleanly wash in water. Dry them in the sun and pound into fine powder. Put the powder in a retort, pour 30 srs. clear water, close up the mouth and apply heat. When half the water has boiled over, remove it from fire. Now collect otto from the distillate.

According to a more convenient method boil down 30 srs. of water until 10 srs. have evaporated. Put the pounded *Khus* roots in an earthen vessel and pour the boiled water over them. Leave it in an open space. After 7 or 8 days a scum will arise on the surface. Soak the froth with cotton and put in a stoppered phial. Place it for a month in the sun and in dew at night to clarify. Finally pack in stoppered phials.

JANTI

Procedure: Take half seer of stalked *Janti* flowers and put in a wide-mouthed bottle. Pour into it 2 srs. good sandal oil. Close the mouth and place in the sun and in dew for 24 hours. Then squeeze the soaked flowers and immerse in the oil a fresh lot of half seer flowers. Close the mouth and place in the sun and in dew for 24 hours. Repeat the process for 16 times replacing the soaked flowers by fresh ones. Finally press.

PUMELO

Procedure: Take 3 srs. of *Pumelo* flowers free from stalks, put them in a wide-mouthed bottle. Pour into it ½ sr. sandal oil, close up the mouth and place for a month in the sun and in dew at night. Press out the oil, store in a stoppered phial and place in the sun for a month to clarify. The flowers must be freshly blown and not in bud.

SHEPHALICA

Procedure: Take 4 ch. stalked *Shephalica* flowers, put in a vessel and pour over them half seer sandal oil. Cover up and set aside for 24 hours. Filter through a funnel. Put the otto again into the vessel and soak into it a fresh lot of 2 ch. flowers. Repeat the process 10 times. Thereby a concentrated otto will be obtained. Finally clarify by placing for one month in the sun and in dew at night.

SANDALWOOD

I

Procedure: A large globular clay pot, with a circular mouth, about 2½ feet deep by about 6 feet circumference at the bulge is taken. The mouth of the pot is closed with a clay lid having a small hole in its centre, through which a bent copper tube about 5½ feet long is passed for the escape of the vapour. The lower end of the tube is conveyed inside a copper receiver, placed in a large porous vessel containing cold water. For preparation of the sandalwood oil, the white or sapwood is rejected, and the heart-wood is cut into small chips, of which about 25 seers or 50 lbs. are put into the pot. As much water is then added as will just cover the chips, and the distillation is carried on slowly for 10 days and nights, by which time the whole of the oil is extracted. As the water from time to time gets low in the still, fresh supplies are added from the heated contents of the refrigerator. The yield of the oil by the above process is said to average 2.5 per cent.

II

Procedure: Reduce the sandalwood to fine powder by filing, and soak the powder in water for 48 hours, before placing it in a copper still tinned inside. Change the receivers directly they are full, return the watery layer of the distillate at certain intervals to the still, and continue the distillation for about a week day and night, maintaining a uniform heat and observing the utmost cleanliness. The above method of distillation requires a high consumption of fuel.

The modern method of distillation would not only reduce the cost of production but also increase the percentage of yield of the oil. The plant required has to be of special design consisting of the following:

1. A rasping machine, with which to comminute the sandal wood into fine filing.

2. An efficient form of steam still complete with tubular condenser, Florentine flasks, etc.

3. A small copper still for re-distillation of the oil.

4. A boiler capable of generating super-heated steam.

ARTIFICIAL OTTOS

Ottos are being gradually replaced by cheap foreign synthetic perfumes. Some otto manufacturers have resorted to the practice of adding aromatic chemicals to their blends with a view to cheapen the cost to enable them to compete with the perfume compounds from Europe. It is evident that the taste in India is being more and more influenced by Western blends.

Artificial ottos are prepared from artificial sources, mainly from heiko scents. A typical recipe follows:

To prepare Otto *Bela* take Heiko *Bela* 2 oz. and Sandal Oil 8 oz. Mix together and keep aside for 15 days.

MARKETING

The otto preparations should be perfectly clear and free from turbidity. The phials should be perfectly dried before the ottos are poured into them as the presence of moisture tends to separate the aromatics.

The glass phials must have ground glass stoppers in place of cork stoppers which due to the presence of cork impart a peculiar odour. To exclude air the stoppers are covered down to the bottle necks with capsules of animal membrane.

SECTION FOUR
AROMATIC WATERS

CHAPTER XII

ROSE AND KEORA WATER

ROSE WATER AND OTTO

The rose principally cultivated in this country for the manufacture of rose water is the Damask Rose (Rose Damascena), otherwise known as Bashra or Persian Rose.

The flowers are plucked early in the morning and conveyed in large bags to the distillers. The apparatus for distilling is of the simplest description; it consists of a large copper or iron boiler, well tinned, capable of holding from 8 to 12 gallons with a large body, a rather narrow neck, and a mouth about 8 inches in diameter, on the top of which is fixed the head of the still. This is merely a *dekchi* with a hole in the bottom to receive the tube of water which is well luted with flour and water. This tube is composed of two pieces of bamboo fastened together at an acute angle and covered in their whole length with a coating of string, over which mud is luted to prevent the vapour from escaping. The lower end of the tube is carried down into a long-necked vessel or receiver, called a *bhubka*. This is kept in a *handi* of water, which as it gets hot is changed. The end of the tube in the *bhubka* is padded with cloth to keep in the vapour. The boiler is let into an earthen furnace, and after being charged with the roses and a sufficient quantity of water, distillation is slowly proceeded with. A boiler of the size described will hold about 10,000 roses; about 10 seers of water will be poured on these flowers, and 8 seers of rose water will be obtained. After distillation, the rose water is placed in a glass carboy and exposed to the sun for several days to become ripe, after which the mouth is stoppered with cotton over which a covering of moist clay is put to prevent the scent from escaping.

To procure the attar, after the rose-water has been distilled, it is placed in a large metal basin which is covered with wetted muslin to prevent dust and insects from getting in; this vessel is then let into the ground which has been previously wetted with water and allowed to remain there during the whole night. While it cools a little film of *attar* forms on the surface of the rose water which is removed in the morning by means of a feather and placed in a small phial, and day after day, as the collection is made, it is placed for a short time in the sun, and after a sufficient quantity has been procured, it is poured off clear into small phials. The first few days' distillation does not produce such fine *attar* as is obtained afterwards, since it is mixed with dust and particles of dirt from the still. It has been calculated that one tola of *attar* is produced from one lakh of roses approximately. More, however, may be obtained if the roses are full-sized and the nights cool enough to allow of the coagulation. The rose water should always be distilled twice, the water procured from the first distillation being used to pour over the roses for the second one.

Distillation may however be dispensed with in preparing rose water as the following recipes will show:

I

Rose	5 seers
Clear Water	10 seers

Procedure: First put the cleaned rose petals in an earthen vessel. Next heat the water in another earthenware vessel. Then pour the boiling water on to the petals and close up the containing vessel so that air is excluded. Strain after one hour and the filtrate will be good rose water to serve all purposes.

II

Rose Petals	5 seers
Water	10 seers

Procedure: Put in an earthenware vessel; close the mouth with a plate luted with mud. Apply gentle heat for 3 hours and allow to cool. Strain when cold and the filtrate will be good rose water.

III

Rose Oil	2.5 grams
Clove Oil	0.25 gram
Alcohol to make	100 c.c.
Distilled Water	10,000 c.c.

Procedure: Mix the first two ingredients and add alcohol to make 100 c.c. Now mix the spirituous liquid with 10,000 c.c. of boiling distilled water and allow to stand until it has undergone the viscous fermentation and blend producing a stuff superior to most of the commercial rose water.

The above recipe obviates the necessity of distilling rose petals and yields rose water of satisfactory quality on simply mixing the ingredients mentioned in the recipe.

KEORA WATER

I

Keora flower	100 seers
Water	1 maund

Procedure: Select only the white petals rejecting the green leaves and the pollen. Proceed to distillation as in the case of rose water (page 101). The distiller is a tinned copper or iron boiler having a capacity of 8 to 12 gallons. The boiler is let into an earthen furnace, and charged with Keora flowers and a sufficient quantity of water. Temperature is not allowed to go high and distillation is carried on slowly. After distillation the Keora water is kept for 7 days in sunlight to mature.

II

Keora flower	50 seers
Water	10 seers

Procedure: Select only the white petals, over which pour 10 seers of boiling water and close up the containing vessel so that air is excluded. Set aside for 24 hours. Strain and phial.

III

Keora flower	50 seers
Water	10 seers

Procedure: Put the water in an earthenware vessel and throw in the white petals of Keora. Place the whole in the sun for a week and strain. The filtrate will be good Keora water.

CHAPTER XIII

TOILET WATERS

LAVENDER WATER

I

Essential Oil of English Lavender (Burgoyne)	4	oz.
Otto de Rose (Virgin)	2	dr.
Rectified Spirit	4	bottles

Procedure: Mix together and use after three months.

II

Oil Lavender (Herrings)	3	oz.
Rectified Spirit	3	bottles
Tincture Orris	4	oz.
Otto de Rose	1	dr.

Procedure: Mix together and use after one month.

III

Oil Lavender (Grasse, France)	1	oz.
Essence Ambergris	4	oz.
Eau de Cologne	80	oz.
Rectified Spirit	4	oz.

Procedure: Mix together and use after one month.

IV

Oil of Lavender (English)	4	dr.
Essence of Bergamot	20	minims.
Essence Lemon (or Civet)	20	minims.
Otto de Rose	20	minims.
Essence Ambergris	1	dr.
Rectified Spirit	3	pints

Orange Flower Water	4 oz.
Rose Water	12 oz.
Burnt Alum	20 gr.

Procedure: Shake several times and store away in a cool place. Finally strain through filter paper and phial.

V

Oil Lavender (Burgoyne)	3 dr.
Oil Bergamot	3 dr.
Otto de Rose	5 minims.
Oil Cloves	6 minims.
Musk	2 gr.
Oil of Rosemary (true)	1 dr.
Honey	1 oz.
Benzoic Acid	2 scruples
Rectified Spirit	1 pint.
Distilled Water	3 oz.

Procedure: Mix together and allow to mature for 6 months.

VI

Oil of Lavender (Mitchams)	3 dr.
Oil Bergamot	20 minims.
Oil Neroli	6 minims.
Otto de Rose	6 or 12 minims.
Essence of Civet	8 or 10 minims.
Essence Musk	20 minims.
Rectified Spirit	20 oz.
Orange Flower Water	4 oz.

Procedure: Mix together and shake for several times. Store away in a cool place for 3 months. Strain and use.

Amber Lavender

Oil of Lavender (Eng.)	1 oz.
Essence Amber	6 oz.
Rectified Spirit	1 bottle

Procedure: Mix and use after 1 month.

Lily Lavender

Lily lavender, petunia lavender, etc., may be prepared in the same manner by replacing essence amber by essence lily, petunia, etc.

English Lavender Water

Oil of Lavender (Mitchams)	4 oz.
Rose Water	1 bottle
Magnesium Carbonate	q.s.
Alcohol	3 bottles

Procedure: First macerate the oil of lavender with such a quantity of magnesium carbonate in a stone mortar that the whole mixture is converted into a powdery mass. Now pour the rose water and incorporate the powder well into it. Then strain into a glass jar and add alcohol. Store aside for six months.

Ambergris Lavender Water

Oil Lavender (Mitchams)	8 oz.
Essence Musk	4 oz.
" Ambergris	1½ oz.
Oil Bergamot	1½ oz.
Rectified Spirit	2 gallons.

Procedure: This will yield an excellent Lavender water. To be kept for 3 months to mature.

Eau De Lavender Millefleurs

Oil Lavender (English)	2 oz.
Essence of Bergamot	1 dr.
" Lemon	1 dr.
Otto de Rose	1 dr.
Essence of Millefleurs	1½ oz.
" Ambergris	4 dr.
Rectified Spirit	6 pints

Procedure: Mix and use after 6 months when the water fully matures.

Odoriferous Lavender Water

I

Oil Lavender (Mitchams)	20 oz.
Oil Bergamot (Burgoyne)	5 oz.

Essence Ambergris	4	dr.
Orris Root Poweder	4	oz.
Rectified Spirit	5	gallons

Procedure: Mix together and strain after one month.

II

Alcohol	3750	c.c.
Oil of Lavender	100	grams
Oil of Thyme	10	grams
Tincture of Musk	10	grams
Distilled Water	500	c.c.

Procedure: Dissolve the essential oils in the alcohol and then the musk. Lastly, pour the distilled water. Seal the mouth of the jar or bottle and allow to mature for a month before use.

Florida Water

Oil of	Lavender	½	oz.
"	Bergamot	1	oz
"	Cassia	1	dr.
"	Clove	½	dr.
"	Neroli	½	dr.
Essence of Musk		½	oz.
Alcohol		64	oz.
Cinnamon water to make		80	oz.

Mix in the above order.

Violet Water

Oil of	Sandal	4	dr.
"	Bergamot	4	dr.
"	Rose Geranium	1	dr.
"	Neroli	1	dr.
"	Bitter Almonds	15	drops
Musk		1	gr.
Tincture of Benzoin		4	dr.
Powdered Orris Root		2	dr.
Water		60	oz.
Alcohol		100	oz.

Macerate 30 days and filter. The product is coloured with just a trace of green dye.

EAU DE COLOGNE

I

Oil	Bergamot	1 oz.
”	Lemon	$1/2$ oz.
”	Rosemary	2 dr.
”	Neroli	30 minims.
”	Lavender	4 dr.
”	Orange	2 dr.
Rectified Spirit		2 lbs.

Procedure: The ingredients are mixed with brisk shaking one by one. Set the whole aside in a stoppered vessel for a fortnight and during that period shake the vessel thrice daily at a time. Finally filter and pack.

II

Cardamom minor (seeds)		1 tola
Oil	Neroli	14 minims.
”	Citron	14 minims.
”	Bergamot	14 minims.
”	Rosemary	14 minims.
Spirit		1 bottle

Procedure: - Proceed as in I.

III

Otto of	Orange Flower	1 dr.
Oil	Orange	1 oz.
”	Lemon	1 oz.
Essence	Cedrat	4 dr.
Oil	Rosemary	4 dr.
”	Lavender	2 dr.
Spirit		1 bottle

Procedure: Proceed as in I.

IV

Oil	Neroli	30 minims.
”	Orange	1 dr.

Oil	Lemon	1	dr.
Oil	Rosemary	30	minims.
Essence	Bergamot	4	dr.
Spirit		20	oz.

Procedure: Proceed as in I.

V

Oil	Neroli	2½	dr.
"	Lavender	30	minims.
"	Orange	50	minims.
"	Rosemary	40	minims.
"	Lemon	4	dr.
"	Bergamot	1	oz.
Spirit		1	bottle

Procedure: Proceed as in I.

SECTION FIVE
HAIR OIL AND TOILET PREPARATIONS

CHAPTER XIV

SCENTED HAIR OILS

People are quite justified in paying unusual attention to the choice of the oils for dressing the hairs for toileting and before bathing. All readers of beauty admit that the hairs add grace to the appearance. But unless proper care is exercised in selecting the hair oils, the hairs are liable to fall off and turn prematurely grey. A hair oil preparation of the ideal type should add a lustre to the hairs, retain them soft and flowing, invigorate their growth, prevent premature greyness, keep the brain cool and yet should not be sticky at all. It should also possess, if possible a mild perfume. But none of the oils ordinarily met with from vegetable or mineral sources can claim all these properties. Hence the hair oils specially prepared for the purpose and perfumed slightly are in ever-increasing demand.

POPULARITY OF HAIR OILS

Enormous popularity of all sorts of hair oils should, therefore, warrant the careful attention of all perfumers. The field before them, so far as the manufacture of hair oil is concerned, is absolutely limitless. In fact a good number of preparations commanding big sales in the market can hardly claim to be good and non-injurious. In the face of these facts one is emboldened to say that any really good preparation delightfully perfumed has a bright future before it.

Mention may be made at the outset that in contrast with the manufacture of floral oils, the perfumers will find the preparation of scented hair oils a relatively tame affair. No elaborate process are to be undergone. The difficulties of raw materials are not insuperable and the scents and essential oils which largely enter into the composition of hair oils are available at all seasons. Only what is necessary are scrupulous care and careful manipulation throughout the operations.

CHIEF CONSTITUENTS

The scented hair oils mostly have some oil or combination of oils as their basis and suitable perfumes are added in proper quantities to produce a pleasant refreshing odour. It should be distinctly understood that the nature of the scents to be introduced should be governed no less by the base oil than by the popular taste. Moreover, some fixative agents should be present in the preparation to bind down the fragrance so that this may not disappear after a few hours and even on bathing. The more the perfume persists, the superior is the quality of the oil, no doubt.

BASE OILS

The oils more generally employed as basis in the manufacture of ordinary hair oils are of vegetable origin such as castor oil, coconut oil and til or sesamum oil. There are other oils as well of vegetable origin like mustard oil, olive oil, groundnut oil, suitable for the making of hair oils, but their use for the purpose is rather restricted, though groundnut oil is coming into favour for cheapness and adulteration.

VEGETABLE BASE OILS

Castor oil, coconut oil and sesamum oil continue to be the most used, either alone or in combination with others to supplement their individual properties and to counter-balance the defects. Castor oil, for example, stimulates growth of hairs and is a most useful agent where hair-enriching aspect of the hair oil is desired to be attained. But it has got one drawback. It is of thick consistency and unless very finely refined it is liable to cause uneasy stickiness of hairs. Hence rarely castor oil is employed alone as a base oil though it is present in prescribed quantities in many oil preparations of the superior type.

Coconut oil is in all respects an ideal base oil in summer; it softens the hairs, imparts a lustre, is of thin consistency and does not cause stickiness. But one unsurmountable defect from which it suffers is that the oil solidifies in the cold season. The freeziness is however prevented by the addition of other base oils, such as sesamum, castor and even mineral oils. One part of coconut oil in mixture with three parts of other oils will be an ideal oil base.

Sesamum oil is thicker than coconut oil and thinner than castor oil. This can be used alone as an oil base. The oil keeps the brain cool but long use renders the hairs sticky and sometimes retards the growth of hairs.

MINERAL BASE OILS

Oils of mineral origin are also used in the making of hair oils. The most commonly known of them is the white oil. The oil is very thin but its use in hair oil making is very restricted as this is directly injurious to the hairs. The great fluidity of the oil is a great asset and if this is to be used at all, its evil effects are to be counter-balanced by the admixture of suitable oil bases and essential oils. Of late, its use has expanded for hair oil making for its cheapness, whiteness and fluidity, and even somtimes contrary to the first elements of hygiene, it is used alone for ensuring cheapness. In general, however, preference should be extended to vegetable oils to mineral oils.

BENZOATED OILS

Benzoated oils are sometimes used as basis in the preparation of hair oils. These do not get rancid with age and help preserving the scents incorporated into the oils.

Essentially benzoated oils are made by digesting 1 oz. of bruised benzoin in a pint of sweet or olive oil for 3 hours on a water bath and filtering through filter paper. Detailed method follows:

Heat on a water bath 1,000 parts of vegetable oil and when hot add to this 100 parts of powdered sodium bicarbonate. Stir and when the bicarbonate gets dissolved, add 100 parts of benzoic acid. In some cases benzoin is added in place of benzoic acid but in this case benzoin 100 parts in weight should first be enclosed in a cheese cloth bag and is then suspended in the oil. This concentrated benzoated oil is to be diluted with vegetable oils before use in hair oils. Usually 1 part of this is mixed with 20 parts of vegetable oil and 1 part of terpeneol to mask the oily odour.

FLORAL OILS IN HAIR OIL MAKING

There is another class of base oil used in making hair oils, we mean the floral oils. These are employed in the manufacture of the superior kinds of the hair oils. *Bela* oil, *Chameli* oil, *henna* oil, etc., are however the most employed. The oils by themselves possess a most delicate fragrance which is further mildly modified by the addition of choicest perfumes. These constitute one of the best base oils. They are thin, keep the hair soft and brain cool, do not cause stickiness; but one way they are defective, they do not—in spite of their sweet perfume—help the growth of hair and as a matter of fact retard its growth and on long use the hairs grow less dense and fall off. This defect can, however, be remedied by the introduction of balsam Peru, cantharidin and fly cantharides which are all highly recommended by the physicians as the agents that invigorate the growth of hairs and prevent baldness.

INCORPORATION OF PERFUMES

Next in importance to the oil bases in making hair oils is the perfume. Extreme care should be taken in the selection of the scents, which are mostly essential oils derived from natural and sometimes from synthetic sources to cheapen the cost of production. More than one perfuming agent is made use of and their combination is effected in judicious sequence by careful manipulation. The scents are to be incorporated in prescribed quantities, for too much of one scent may spoil the harmonious character of the final aroma. The scents, moreover, should not be fugitive. To gain this end sandal oil and other fixative agents are called into requisition, as already referred to.

MANIPULATIONS

In manufacturing hair oils, due attention should be concentrated on the manipulations. Good and fresh raw materials of course go far towards the preparation of excellent hair oils but without methodical manipulations the perfumer, with the best of materials and intentions, will fail to produce hair oils of real worth.

FILTRATION AND REFINING

First, the vegetable oils ordinarily used in the preparation of hair oils require to be refined thoroughly and freed from suspended impurities. A beginner in the line can purchase refined oils from the market but as a matter of fact big manufacturers find it more expedient to refine the oils themselves. This saves cost and helps to increase the profits. Specially the castor oil and sesamum oil should be in a highly refined state if the consistency is to be thinned down and the stickiness of the oil is to be removed.

Oridinarily it is the custom with the perfumer to filter the oil. The task of filtration is rather tedious and the operation requires a long time for completion but nevertheless the operation is most necessary. The operation should be allowed to proceed on without haste. To expedite the matter several jars may be fitted with funnels for filtration. When the oil is once filtered, it will be often found that it is not sufficiently purified for use in hair oils. In such cases the operation of filtration is repeated several times.

FILTRATION OF THICK OILS

Filtration of thick oils is however attended with great difficulties as the oil only comes down in drops at long intervals. In such cases the oil may be strained through good flannel, two or three times. The flannel may be made two-fold or three-fold to get better results. Sometimes with the same end in view, the flannel is fitted into big funnels and oils are poured into them for filtration.

REFINING WITH ANIMAL CHARCOAL.

Straining through flannel and filtration will often be found sufficient but in some cases, specially in the matter of castor oil, the oil may be refined more efficiently, cheaply and completely with the help of animal charcoal. Animal charcoal, it may be pointed out, is made by first boiling bones with water so as to remove gelatine and then by heating in iron retorts.

As soon as the process of distillation is finished, the solid residue is transferred into iron containers whose mouths are instantly closed air-tight and allowed to cool. The carbonised bones are then ground in a mill and sorted by sieves into 2 grades. The finely powdered product is known as ivory black while the coarse powder goes by the name of animal charcoal. The charcoal is spread in layers in a wide vessel and the oil to be refined is slowly introduced into it. The mouth of the vessel is then covered up to prevent dust, dirt and sand from coming in contact with the oil. The whole is then put in the sun for a fortnight and is thus completely bleached.

To refine oil with animal charcoal use may be made of a percolator which is a cylindrical vessel with fine perforations at the bottom. It is placed on a stand below which is placed a receptacle for collecting any liquid, dropping through the perforations. The false bottom of the percolator is covered with a layer of powder and dried animal charcoal twelve to fifteen inches in thickness. The oil to be refined is gently poured over the bed of charcoal and left to work its way through the same by gravity. During descent, the oil gives up its colour and odour to the charcoal with which it comes into contact. The process of percolation may be repeated till a point is reached when the percolating oil viewed in a layer one inch in thickness cannot be distinguished from clear water but would have a pale colour in a sufficiently thick layer.

The process is necessarily a slow one but it needs no attention and can be continued day and night. For a large outturn the dimensions of the percolator may be suitably increased, or better, a series of percolators may be used.

When the charcoal loses its power of absorbing colour and odour after use for some time, it requires revivification.

Chemical processes have now been evolved for bleaching oils but these are complex and require elaborate machineries and expert scientific knowledge. There are other methods of refining oils, for details of which refer to *page* 21. For the perfumery manufacturer the method of refining with animal charcoal will be the easiest and at the same time the best. Actually by such treatment raw castor oil No. 3 can be turned into oil No. 1 without any trouble.

COCONUT OIL REFINING

A special process of refining coconut oil for hair oils has lately been worked out at the Harcourt Butler Technological Institute, Cawnpore which is given below:

The process consists in boiling for a few hours the sample of coconut oil with a 2 per cent solution of sodium silicate, removing the soap formed and finally washing and drying the oil. The weight of sodium silicate used for a given quantity of oil depends upon the free fatty acid content of the oil and the alkalinity of the silicate. The quantity of sodium silicate taken is such that its alkalinity is exactly equivalent to the acidity of the oil. Usually with an oil of 3 per cent acidity, the quantity of sodium silicate of 140^0 Tw. required is 1.6 lb. per 100 lbs. of the oil.

The oil, taken in a vessel with a tapering bottom and a stop-cock, is heated to about 80^0C and its equivalent of 2 per cent silicate solution previously warmed to about 50^0C is poured slowly into it with vigorous stirring. The heating is continued for some time till the liquid comes to boiling. Then as the boiling goes on, water is poured in from time to time to make up for the loss by evaporation and this is continued for about two and and half hours. By this time the issuing steam is found to have hardly any odour of coconut oil.

At this stage, about 5 lbs. of powdered common salt are added, and the whole boiled for a few minutes to coagulate the soap formed. The liquid is then allowed to stand, and the emulsion of soap and silicic acid is carefully drawn off from the bottom. The residual oil is given two or three washings with hot water, till the wash liquid no longer gives any alkaline reaction. After every washing the wash water is drawn off from the bottom. The washed oil is then heated in a shallow dish with constant stirring to drive off any residual moisture.

The oil may finally be mixed with 1 per cent "diatomite earth" and filtered, when the oil becomes perfectly clear, bright and without any perceptible odour.

Another easy process of refining coconut oil follows:

In order to prepare scented coconut oil, the oil is to be deodorised first. For this purpose take 100 tolas of coconut oil in a suitable vessel. Then weigh out 1 tola of 98 per cent caustic soda and dissolve it in 10 tolas of water. Now warm the oil over a water bath and stir in 2½ tolas of the alkali solution as prepared above. Continue warming for a few minutes and then sprinkle 1 tola of salt. Stir vigorously for some time and skim off about 5 tolas of scum by means of a ladle. Then remove the oil from the water bath and set aside to cool. Next filter the oil and put it in the sun after covering the vessel with a piece of clean cloth to protect it from being contaminated with dust. By this means any moisture present in the oil is evaporated.

The oil thus prepared is practically odourless.

DEODORISING COCONUT OIL

Two methods are well known for the deodorisation of coconut oil:

1. Wash out the odoriferous bodies with alcohol. This removes the fatty acids, and also such substances as phytostero. Some employ a joint process of washing with alcohol followed by treatment with animal charcoal.

2. Pass high pressure steam at 6-8 atmosphere into the fluid oil for two or three hours; the non-volatile fatty acids left are to be removed by adding 0.25 per cent of calcined magnesia, and the magnesium soap formed as a result of this is then skimmed off the surface.

(3) The odour of raw coconut oil may be masked to some extent by the addition of lemongrass oil or citronella oil.

The oil is however likely to develop bad odour again unless special care is taken to store the oil in a convenient place. Any contact with moist air engenders rancidity of the oil.

REFINING CASTOR OIL

The refining of crude castor oil consists mainly in the removal of the albumen, free fatty acids, colouring and odorous matters, and is conducted by first coagulating the albuminous matter and mucilage by steaming and filtering, then bleaching and deodorising by agitation in the presence of animal charcoal, and finally filtering and drying. The bleaching of the solvent extracted castor oil has been found to be a difficult operation. The colouring matter is held in colloidal suspension and has probably become very firmly fixed during the heating operation. It is most resistant to the action of bleaching agent.

I

The process of refining castor oil consists in treating the oil with animal charcoal in the proportion of four to one by weight.

Animal charocoal should be finely ground before it is mixed to the crude oil. The whole is put in glass or China jars and covered over with a lid and is then exposed to the rays of the sun for 15 days successively. Impurities are absorbed by the charcoal and on filtering refined oil is obtained.

Use may be made in this connection as in the case of bleaching coconut oil of a percolator which is cylindrical vessel with fine perforations at the bottom. It is placed on a stand, below which is placed a receptacle for collection any liquid, dropping through the perforations. The false bottom of the percolator is covered with a layer of powdered and dried animal charcoal twelve to fifteen inches in thickness. The oil to be refined is gently poured over the bed of charcoal and left to work its way through the same by gravity. During descent, the oil gives up its colour and odour to the charcoal with which it comes into contact. The process of percolation may be repeated till a point is reached when the percolating oil viewed in a layer one inch in thickness would have a pale colour.

The process is necessarily a slow one but it needs no attention and can be continued day and night. For a large output the dimension of the percolator may be suitably increased, or better, a series of percolators may be used.

When the charcoal loses its power of absorbing colour and odour after use for some time, it requires revivification.

II

To clarify castor oil mix 100 parts of the oil at 95°F, with a mixture of 1 part of alcohol (96 per cent) and 1 part of sulphuric acid. Allow to settle for 24 hours and then carefully decant from the precipitate. Now wash with warm water; boiling for ½ hour, allow to settle for 24 hours in well closed vessels, after which the time the purified oil may be taken off.

III

Oil	20 parts
Bichromate of potash	2 parts
Sulphuric acid	3 parts

Dissolve the bichromate in hot water, add the acid, then slowly put this mixture into the oil, agitating, if possible with hot air, or, if this cannot be done, a rouser made of lead may be used. It should nearly fit the bottom of the tub, and be perforated with as many holes as possible. It must be worked up and down either by hand, or fitted to a mechanical stirrer, till the oil becomes pale green. Separate the oil from the chemicals and add half per cent oxalic acid with boiling water, agitate all the time till oil becomes clear, bright and odourless.

DEODORISAING CASTOR OIL

Deodorisation of castor oil may be effected according to any of the following processes:

I

Deodorising of castor oil may be effected by subjecting it to the simultaneous action of steam at 108°C to 110°C, and of a saturated situation of alum or aluminium sulphate. The oil is kept at a temperature of about 80°C until the sediments deposit, after which the clear upper layer, which is now odourless, is withdrawn.

II

Charge 1 ton of oil in an open tank, turn on steam, and when at 120°F, stir in chloride of lime 19 lbs., animal charcoal 2 lbs., black oxide of manganese 28 lbs., and water 7 gallons. As soon as the oil is heated, add 25 lbs. hydrochloric acid, then add 20 lbs. sulphuric acid diluted in 1 gallon water, and boil slowly for 40 minutes. Turn off steam, allow to settle, and, when cold, it will be found to be free from smell.

REFINING GROUNDNUT OIL

The groundnut oil as expressed from the seed is liable to contain mucilage and albuminous matters, which produce turbidity in the oil. In order to remove these impurities, filter the oil through a filter press; but before doing so treat the oil with 10 per cent of its weight of fuller's earth, which should be dehydrated by roasting prior to use. Mix thoroughly and then heat the mixture to 100°F, and maintain the temperature constant for about 15 minutes. Lastly filter the oil through filter press. Thus a clear oil is obtained but the odour of the oil is somewhat earthy. To remove this bad odour wash the oil with 1 per cent solution of brine containing an equal amount of dry sodium bicarbonate.

BLEACHING GROUNDNUT OIL

Treatment of oil with fuller's earth, not only helps to bleach the groundnut oil but also assists in deodorising it to a certain extent.

The principle underlying the process is to mix the fuller's earth intimately with the oil to be treated and subsequently to remove from the oil the fuller's earth together with oil suspended matter. Heat, it has been found, quickens coagulation. The oil is thereby rendered clear and bright.

To ensure almost through incorporation of fuller's earth in the body of the oil, use is made of a mixing kettle which is used jacketed on the bottom only but is occasionally jacketed either partly or completely over the cylindrical surface in addition to the bottom. The additional jacketing may be taken advantage of where there is necessity of maintaining the heat of the kettle for a pretty long time. The kettle is provided with a mechanical agitator and steam coil. A filter press works near the mixing kettle and provision of a pump is made to transfer the batch of treated oil into the filter press in the shortest possible time.

The kettle is first heated by admitting steam to the jacket, care being taken to see that the steam is allowed to blow freely from the outlet provided for draining out the condensed water from the jacket. The oil already heated to a temperature of 150°F, is then run into the kettle until this is filled to within about 4 in. of the top cover; the mixing gear is put to work in the meantime in order to agitate the oil and drive off any moisture contained therein.

The successful working of the process depends to a considerable extent upon the complete absence of moisture, and it is essential, therefore, that the oil, fuller's earth, filter cloths, etc., and the whole of the apparatus should be as dry as possible. The fuller's earth is added as soon as the oil in the kettle is at a temperature of about 150°F. It is important that the fuller's earth should be ground to a very fine powder. The quantity of earth necessary usually varies between about 2½ and 5 per cent but it may be more or less according to the quality of the oil or fat being treated. The exact proportion can be determined by an experiment on a small scale. The experimental test will also enable the most suitable temperature to be ascertained.

It is advisable that the process should be worked at the minimum temperature found to give the required result, as there is less danger of earthy flavour being imparted to the oil at a lower temperature. After a few minutes' agitation the earth will be uniformly and intimately mixed throughout the whole of the oil, and the feed pump on the filter press should then be started to work, and the whole batch pumped into the filter press in the shortest possible time. As soon as the filtering operation is finished, the fuller's earth remaining in the filter press, should be steamed out in order to recover as much as possible of the oil contained in the earth. This is done by opening the steam valve on the head of the filter press and allowing live steam to blow through as quickly as possible until the oil ceases to flow from the outlets of the plates. It is most important that the steam be as dry as possible, and to this end a drain cock should be fitted on the steam pipe just before it enters the filter press, and the steam pipe thoroughly drained out immediately before steaming out the press.

Immediately after steaming out, the press must be opened and the plates separated from each other, so as to leave an equal space between all the plates. If this is done, the heat contained in the iron plates will dry the cloths and deposit fuller's earth on same, so that the fuller's earth can be readily removed from the cloths without taking them off the plates, and will in this way leave the cloths quite clean and ready for a fresh charge.

ADDITION OF SCENTS

The addition of the perfumes also must be methodical. Haphazard methods cannot lead to successful preparations. They should be added one after another in the order they are put in the recipes. The order should not be changed by any means. Moreover a few minutes' time should be allowed to the fixation of one scent before the next one is incorporated and if possible the whole mass should be agitated carefully so that the scent may be intimately incorporated, absorbed by the oil itself and sweetly tempered. After the whole preparation is finished, the mass is recommended to be set aside for a certain period of time before final bottling. This is a most important matter that should not be overlooked by the manufacturers. It is found that on keeping the preparation substantially improves in quality, and hence whenever excellent quality is desired to be attained, the preparation should be allowed to stand for a number of days before final packing.

COLOURING HAIR OILS

The coloration of the hair oils is not a difficult affair. For red, the alkanet root is mostly in vogue. This is cheap and being of vegetable origin is perfectly non-injurious. For yellow shade saffron may be added but this is rarely done as this is rather costly. Now-a-days all tints in hair oils except red are produced by the incorporation of aniline dyes. But from hygienic point of view these are not non-injurious to health and their use should be as much restricted as permissible.

MARKETING

Finally in marketing the hair oils, decent phials should be used. These should be nicely corked and capsuled and labelled and put in decent cardboard boxes.

RECIPES

A few typical recipes for making scented hair oils follow:

I

Refined Coconut or Sesamum Oil	5	seers
Balsam Peru	2½	oz.
Fly Cantharides	5	dr.
Sandal Oil	15	dr.
Alkanet Root	15	dr.
Otto of Henna	5	dr.
Oil Rosemary	10	dr.

Procedure: First of all the oil is treated with alkanet root and allowed to remain undisturbed for 2 days for colouring. Then strain the oil through cloth. The fly cantharides are next fried in about one chhatak of fresh coconut or sesamum oil and when these are well fried and discoloured, these are allowed to cool. Afterwards add the previously coloured oil, and the Balsam Peru (after melting it over a slow fire). Finally add the other ingredients one by one with constant shaking.

II

Bela Oil		24	oz.
Alkanet Root		2	dr.
Oil	Lavender	2	dr.
"	Geranium Gaul	4	dr.
"	Cloves	1 dr. 26	minims.
"	Cinnamon	1 dr. 46	minims.
"	Bergamot	4	dr.

Procedure: The bela oil of the finest make is first treated with alkanet root and allowed to remain undisturbed for two days together. Strain the oil through a fine cloth when coloured oil will be obtained. To this then add oil lavender and agitate well for 15 minutes; next add the oil geranium and shake again for 15 minutes. Similarly, add the other ingredients one after another and shake the whole for 15 minutes each time. When all the ingredients are added, keep the whole aside air-tight for 15 days, then it will be ready for packing and use.

III

Refined	Sesamum Oil	24	oz.
Alkanet	Root	2	dr.
Oil	Bergamot	6	dr.
"	Lemon	3	dr.
"	Rosemary	2	dr.
"	Neroli	1	dr.
"	Lavender (English)	2	dr.
"	Orange	1	dr.
"	Rose Geranium	2	dr.
Cantharidin		3	grains
Balsam Peru		2	dr.

Procedure: The best quality of refined sesamum oil is taken and into it is added 2 dr. of alkanet root previously cut into small pieces. The whole is then allowed to stand undisturbed for 2 days and then filtered through a piece of fine cloth. Next add the other ingredients one after another in the order they appear in the recipe and shake the whole for 15 minutes after each such addition. Balsam Peru, the last ingredient, is to be melted over a slow fire before incorporation. When the ingredients are all incorporated, the whole is kept aside air-tight in a vessel for a fortnight and then packed.

IV

Chameli Oil	48 oz.
Flora Jasmine	4 dr.
Heiko White Rose	2 dr.
Oil Neroli	1 dr.
” Bergamot	2 dr.
” Lavender	1 dr.
Otto Pimento	30 minims.
Heiko Amber	2 dr.
Oil of Cantharides	1 oz.
Alkanet Root	4 dr.

Procedure: Only the superior quality of *Chameli* oil should be taken for making good hair oils. This is then treated with the alkanet roots broken into small fragments and left aside undisturbed for 2 days. Finally strain and add the other ingredients one after another with constant shaking. Next allow the oil to remain in a vessel air-tight for 7 days. Finally strain and pack into phials.

V

Chameli Oil	2 seers
Almond Oil	1 seer
Alkanet Root	1 oz.
Cantharidin	12 grains
Balsam Peru	5 oz.
Sandal Oil	3 oz.
Flora Jasmine	12 dr.
English Lavender	2 oz.

Procedure: Mix the *Chameli* and almond oil together and drop into this the alkanet root in small pieces and let the oil remain undisturbed for 2 days. Then strain through a piece of cloth and add the ingredients one after another with constant shaking. While adding the balsam peru take care that it is melted over a slow fire before addition. When all the ingredients are well incorporated, pack in a vessel with the mouth well-covered and put in the strong sunlight for 20 days together. Finally strain and pack into phials.

This oil helps the growth of hair and prevents baldness.

VI

Castor Oil	3 seers
Alkanet Root	1 oz.
Tincture Cantharidin	4 dr.
Oil Rosemary (True)	1 oz.
English Lavender	1 oz.
Heiko Tuberose	1 oz.

Procedure: Alkanet root is first of all added into the castor oil in small fragments and then put in strong sunlight for 20 days together and strained through a fine cotton cloth. The other ingredients are then added one after another with constant shaking. Allow the whole to remain undisturbed for 7 days together. Finally strain again and pack into phials.

This oil invigorates the growth of hair and prevents baldness.

VII

Sesamum Oil	6 seers
Alkanet Root	2 oz.
Otto Keora	1 oz.
Oil Lavender	2 oz.
" Rosemary	1 oz.

Procedure: The sesamum oil is first of all treated with animal charcoal and put in the sun for a fortnight. This is then filtered through a filter paper or through flannel. To the oil thus refined add the alkanet root in small bits and strain after two days. Then incorporate the other ingredients one after another with constant stirring and let the whole stand for 7 days in a vessel tightly corked. Finally strain again and pack into phials.

This oil keeps the brain cool and stimulates the growth of hair.

VIII

Sesamum Oil		1½ seers.
Alkanet	Root	4 dr.
Heiko	Cananga	1 oz.
Oil	Lavender	1 oz.
"	Verbena	1 oz.
"	Sandal	1 oz.

Procedure: The sesamum oil is first of all refined by treating it with animal charcoal and allowing the whole to lie in strong sunlight for 15 days together. The oil is then filtered through flannel and into this the alkanet roots are added in small bits. Then whole is again set aside for 2 days and then filtered. Next add the other ingredients one after another with constant stirring and leave the whole undisturbed in a vessel closely corked. Finally strain once again and pack.

The oil is delicious, non-sticky and keeps the brain cool.

IX

Coconut	Oil	12 ch.
White	Oil	4 ch.
Oil	Lavender	3 dr.
"	Sandal	3 dr.
Oil	Bergamot	3 dr.
Alkanet	Root	1½ dr.

Procedure: First refine the coconut oil and add the alkanet roots. The whole is left for colouring for 2 days. Now filter and add the essential oils one by one and shake well before the addition of the next one. The whole is left well corked for 7 days for ripening, then phial.

X

White	Oil	24 oz.
Sesamum	Oil	12 oz.
Coconut	Oil	6 oz.
Castor	Oil	6 oz.
Alkanet	Root	4 dr.
Orris	Root Powder	8 dr.

Rose Otto	1 tollah
Oil of Neroli	2 dr.
" Lavender	8 dr.

Procedure: Orris root in a powdered condition and bruised alkanet root are introduced into the mixture of the oils. The whole is then put in the sun for a fortnight. Filter and to the clear oil add the essential oils one by one, shaking the vessel well before adding the next one.

XI

Coconut Oil	4 oz.
Castor Oil	3 oz.
White Oil	7 oz.
Oil of Lavender	1 dr.
" Bergamot	30 minims
" Rose Geranium	10 oz.
Alkanet Root	1¼ dr.

Procedure : - Mix the oils and treat with the alkanet root. After 3 days, filter and add the essential oils one by one, shaking the bottle each time for a few minutes.

XII

Castor Oil	15 oz.
Alcohol	3 oz.
Oil of Nutmeg	30 minims.
" Rosemary	10 minims.
" Sweet Marjoram	10 minims.
" Neroli	10 minims.
Oil of Rose	20 minims.
Tincture of Musk	1 dr.
Alkanet Root	q.s.

Procedure: Mix the castor oil with alcohol and colour with sufficient amount of alkanet root. Filter and incorporate the essential oils one by one shaking briskly each time for a little while.

XIII

Sesamum Oil	1,000 parts
Lavender Oil	12 parts

Lemon Oil	20 parts
Rosemary Oil	5 parts
Geranium Oil	2 parts

Procedure: Colour the oil suitably and add the scents one by one. This gives a cheap preparation.

XIV

Til, Coconut or Castor oil	500 parts
Balsam Peru	15 parts
Oil of Jasmine	60 parts
" of Roses	30 parts
" of Bitter Almonds	30 parts
" of Vanilla	60 parts
" of Ambergris	30 parts
" of Musk	30 parts

Procedure: The balsam Peru is first of all digested for 14 days in the oil, shaking the vessel frequently. When the mixture is clear, add the essential oils one by one. The oil keeps for a long time and resembles very much the heliotrope oil in odour.

XV

Sesamum Oil	8 ch.
Otto of Roses	50 minims.
Oil of Rosemary	25 minims.
Alkanet Root	1½ dr.

Procedure: Soak the alkanet root in the oil till the desired shade of colour is acquired. Filter and add the scents one by one with shaking for a few minutes in each case.

XVI

Benzoated Oil	20 oz.
Otto of Rose	25 minims.
Heliotropin	20 dr.

Procedure: The benzoated oil is made by digesting an ounce of bruised benzoin, preferably of Siam, in a pint of almond or olive oil for three hours, and filtering through filter paper. Finally add the scent, shake and phial. The oil does not become rancid.

XVII

Deodorised Oil	24 parts

Oil of Orange Blossom	22 parts
" of Jasmine	12 parts
" of Carnation Pinks	1½ parts

Procedure: Mix the whole together by shaking and allow to ripen for a number of days. Phial when the mixture becomes clear.

XVIII

Benzoated Oil	10 oz.
Ionone, 100 per cent	2½ oz.
Otto of Rose	2 minims.
Oil of Jasmine, Syn	3 minims.
" of Cloves	6 minims.
" of Bergamot	12 minims.

Procedure: Mix.

For other odours mix 1 part of any floral oil with 4 parts of benzoated oil.

XIX

Benzoated Oil	10 oz.
Jasmine Oil (floral)	10 dr.
Oil of Cloves	10 drops
" of Bergamot	½ dr.
Otto of Rose	5 drops
Oil of Orange Flower	20 drops
" of Thyme	1 drop

Procedure: Same as in (XVIII).

XX

Refined Coconut Oil	72 oz.
Oil of Rosemary	1 dr.
" of Rose Geranium	1½ dr.
" of Bergamot	½ dr.
Musk Ketone	14 gr.
Benzyl Alcohol	½ dr.

Procedure: Put the coconut oil in a suitable bottle and add to it the essential oils one by one with vigorous shaking. Finally add the musk ketone after dissolving it in benzyl alcohol. Now close the mouth of the bottle with a cork and keep aside for a week before use.

CHAPTER XV

TARAL ALTA

Taral Alta is the Bengali name for a kind of fluid rouge, like lip-salve, for imparting a rosy hue to the skin. It is a universal custom in Bengal and elsewhere amongst Hindu women to paint their feet, palms of hands, finger tips, etc., periodically with indigenous lac dye. This decoration adds to the grace of feminine beauty. And for this purpose the service of the female barber has got to be requisitioned. But with the help of ready-made Taral Alta a lady can paint herself by simply applying the liquid dye with a swab.

Taral Alta is, therefore, now in great vogue. It commands a wide sale specially during marriage season and in times of festivities. Its manufacture will, therefore, be found remunerative.

MODE OF PREPARATION

The mode of preparation of Taral Alta may broadly be divided into two classes. In the first class a chosen essential oil is macerated with magnesium carbonate in a stone mortar with a stone pestle. The mixture is then stirred in distilled water which has been boiled up before use. The emulsion is then filtered through blotting paper. This forms the basic perfumed water to which is dissolved a quantity of scarlet dye, e.g., eosine, rhodamine, crocine scarlet to produce Taral Alta.

A variation of the method consists in soaking freshly blown scented flowers in distilled water in a covered vessel for 24 hours by which time it will absorb their fragrance. The perfumed water is strained through a flannel sheet, and a solution of scarlet dye in this water yields Taral Alta as before.

In any case 1 oz. of methylated spirit may be added to each quart of the products to impart a quick drying property and 1 oz. of powdered gum arabic to ensure a good shine when dry.

MARKETING

The final products should be bottled in decent phials and corked and capsuled. A sponge swab with a wire holder should be inserted in every packet. The label should be printed in attractive design. Instructions should be given first to wash the skin and then to apply uniformly with the swab and finally to allow to dry up.

Rose

A.	Rose Otto	30	minims.
	Magnesium Carbonate	1	oz.
	Distilled Water	12	quarts
B.	Perfumed Water	1	quart
	Scarlet Dye	2	oz.

Procedure: Macerate the essential oil with magnesium carbonate in a stone mortar with a stone pestle. Stir in the distilled water and filter. To the perfumed water thus prepared add the scarlet dye when good scented Alta will be obtained.

Sandal

A.	Sandal Oil	1	tollah
	Magnesium Carbonate	1	oz.
	Distilled Water	6	quarts
B.	Perfumed Water	1	quart
	Scarlet Dye	2	oz.

Procedure: As in Rose Taral Alta.

Lavender

A.	Essential Oil of Lavender (English)	2	dr.
	Magnesium Carbonate	1	oz.
	Distilled Water	3	quarts
B.	Perfumed Water	1	quart
	Scarlet Dye	1	oz.

Procedure: As in Rose Taral Alta.

Lily

A. Heiko Lily
   Magnesium Carbonate — 1 oz.
   Distilled Water — 2 quarts
B. Perfumed Water — 1 quart
   Scarlet Dye — 1 oz.
Procedure: As in Rose Taral Alta.

Henna

A. Henna Otto — 1 tollah
   Magnesium Carbonate — 1 oz.
   Distilled Water — 4 quarts
B. Scarlet Dye — 2 oz.
   Perfumed Water — 2 quarts
Procedure: As in Rose Taral Alta.

Khus

A. Otto of Khus — 1 tollah
   Magnesium Carbonate — 1 oz.
   Distilled Water — 4 quarts
B. Scarlet Dye — 1½ oz.
   Perfumed Water — 2 quarts
Procedure: As in Rose Taral Alta.

Violet

A. Heiko Violet — 4 dr.
   Magnesium Carbonate — 1 oz.
   Distilled Water — 3 quarts
B. Scarlet Dye — 2 oz.
   Perfumed Water — 1 quart
Procedure: As in Rose Taral Alta.

Cherry Laurel

A. Oil of Cherry Laurel — 4 dr.
   Magnesium Carbonate — 1 oz.
   Distilled Water — 2 quarts.
B. Scarlet Dye — 2 oz.
   Perfumed Water — 1 quart.
Procedure: As in Rose Taral Alta.

Tuberose

A.	Tuberoses	4	oz.
	Distilled Water	3	quarts
B.	Perfumed Water	3	"
	Scarlet Dye	4	oz.

Procedure: Soak the flowers in distilled water in a covered vessel for 24 hours and then strain through a piece of flannel. To the perfumed water thus prepared add the prescribed quantity of the scarlet dye.

Bela

A.	Bela Flowers	½	lb.
	Distilled Water	3	quarts
B.	Perfumed Water	1	quart
	Scarlet Dye	1	oz.

Procedure: As in Tuberose Taral Alta.

Jasmine

A.	Jasmine Flowers	4	oz.
	Distilled Water	2	quarts
B.	Perfumed Water	1	quart
	Scarlet Dye	2	oz.

Procedure: As in Tuberose Taral Alta.

Champaka

A.	*Champaka* Flowers	50	
	Distilled Water	2	quarts
B.	Perfumed Water	1	quart
	Scarlet Dye	2	oz.

Procedure: As in Tuberose Taral Alta.

Bakul

A.	Bakul Flowers	5	tollahs
	Distilled Water	2	quarts
B.	Scarlet Dye	2	oz.
	Perfumed Water	1	quart

Procedure: As in Tuberose Taral Alta.

Rose

A.	Petals of Roses of one colour	½	lb.
	Distilled Water	3	quarts
B.	Scarlet Dye	2	oz.
	Perfumed Water	1	quart

Procedure: As in Tuberose Taral Alta.

Ordinary

Rhodamine B Extra	2	oz.
Brilliant crocine	1	oz.
Rectified Spirit	4	oz.
Glycerine	1	lb.
Rose Water	2	oz.
Water	40	oz.

Procedure: Dissolve the colours and glycerine in water and boil. Then set aside to cool. When cold add the spirit and rose water, and bottle.

CHAPTER XVI

TOILET PREPARATIONS

HAIR LOTIONS

Hair lotions have a stimulating effect upon the hair follicles. They are generally perfumed with oil of rosemary as it possesses a good stimulating property.

Cantharides Lotion

Tincture Cantharides	1½ dr.
Aqua Sambuci	11 oz.
Ess. Rosemary (double)	5 dr.

Procedure: Mix and shake well. It will promote the growth of hair.

Millefleurs Lotion

Oil Lavender	3 oz.
Essence Lemon	3 oz.
” Ambergris	4 oz.
Oil Caraway	2 oz.
Rose Water	12 oz.

Procedure: Mix and shake well. To be used after 3 months.

Hungary Lotion

Rectified Spirit	1 pint
Oil of Rosemary	1 oz.
Essence of Ambergris	2 dr.
Rose Water	6 oz.

Procedure: Mix together; shake well; and leave aside for 1 month.

Lavenia Lotion

Rectified Spirit	1 quart
Rose Water	½ pint

Essential Oil of Lemon	$\frac{1}{2}$ oz.
Otto de Rose	15 minims.
Oil of Cloves	30 minims.
" of Neroli	10 minims.

Procedure: Mix the oils in spirit and shake until dissolved. Then add the rose water and allow to mature for about a month.

Odour Delectabilis

Rose Water	4 oz.
Orange Flower Water	4 oz.
Oil of Lavender	1 dr.
" of Cloves	1 dr.
" of Bergamot	2 dr.
Musk artificial	2 gr.
Rectified Spirit	1 pint

Procedure: Mix together and shake until dissolved well. Use after 1 month.

Hair Stimulating Lotion

Cantharidin	0.02 grams
Acetic ether	1 c.c.
Glacial acetic acid	6 c.c.
Bay rum	250 c.c.
Glycerine	50 c.c.
Water to produce	1000 c.c.

Procedure: Dissolve the cantharidin in the acetic ether and add to the bay rum. Then add the other ingredients.

II

Acetum cantharides	15 c.c.
Alcohol	150 c.c
Rosemary oil	15 c.c
Bergamot oil	10 c.c.
Lavender oil	5 c.c.
Rose oil	5 c.c.
Glycerine	50 c.c.
Water to produce	1000 c.c.

III

Quinine Sulphate	2 grams
Tincture of cantharidin	8 c.c.
Eau de Cologne	750 c.c.
Iso-butyl Salicylate	5 c.c.
Orange flower water to produce	1000 c.c.

Procedure: Dissolve the alkaloid in the eau de cologne, add the tincture and the iso-butyl salicylate. Mix the glycerine with 200 c.c. of the water, and add.

IV

Quinine hydrochloride	3 grams
Pilocarpine hydrochloride	1 gram
Lavender water	200 c.c.
Glycerine	20 c.c.
Rose water to produce	1000 c.c.

Procedure: Dissolve the alkaloidal salts in the lavender water and proceed as above. Filter, if necessary.

V

Tincture of cantharidin	5 c.c
Solution of ammonia	50 c.c.
Borax	25 grams
Glycerine	50 c.c
Rosemary Oil	10 c.c.
Alcohol 90 p.c.	125 c.c.
Rosewater	200 c.c.
Orange flower oil	300 c.c.
Water to produce	1000 c.c.

Procedure: Dissolve the oils in the alcohol, and borax in the glycerine and water. Then mix the two solutions and make up to volume with water.

VI

Pilocarpine nitrate	5 grams
Alcohol	90 c.c.

Tincture of cantharidin	10	c.c.
Heliotropin	5	grams
Verbena oil	3	c.c.
Lavender oil	2	c.c.
Glycerine of borax	50	c.c.
Water to produce	1000	c.c.

Procedure: Same as in (V)

LIPSTICKS

Lipsticks are now a universally accepted article of make-up and vary in price very much according to the skill of the manufacturer together with the degree of elegance of the presentation of this cosmetic.

The requirements of a good lipstick are that it must not be injurious, it must spread easily without being excessively greasy; its colour must be reasonably permanent; it must not sweat, crack or crumble. In addition to these requirements, its colour must be absolutely uniform, unchanging and free from mottling.

I

Spermaceti	31	parts
Paraffin	5	parts
Cocoa butter	7	parts
Cholesterin	26	parts
Castor oil	4	parts
Benzoated lard	8.5	parts
Perfume	.9	parts
Benzoic acid	.1	parts
Bromo-acid (acid eosine)	2.5	parts
Butyl stearate	5	parts
Colour	10	parts

Procedure: Dissolve the bromo acid in the butyl stearate, and add the castor oil. Mix the cholesterin and benzoated lard. Add the bromo acid mixture and the colour. Mix thoroughly and run the mass through a mill four times. Then melt the spermaceti, the paraffin and cocoa butter, and add the colour mass. Mix thoroughly and add the perfume and benzoic acid.

When the mass reaches 110°F keep the temperature of the batch at this point while filling the moulds. The best way to do this is to use a small insulated pouring pot which will hold enough to fill one set of moulds. This can be replenished from the main supply from time to time.

Some manufacturers after this procedure melt the waxes and fats together and mix in the colour, bromo acid and perfume. Then they allow the temperature to drop slightly until the batch becomes sufficiently viscous to grind, then the batch is run through the milling rolls several times after which the sticks are moulded. This is an excellent procedure if the milling rolls or mill can be heated, but if a hot mass is run through a cold mill the wax will crystallise and the resulting product will be unsatisfactory.

II

Cocoa butter	5 parts
Cetyl alcohol	3 parts
Stearic acid	4 parts
Paraffin wax	4 parts
Spermaceti	5 parts
White beeswax	21 parts
Lanolin	5.5 parts
Benzoated lard	32 parts
Castor oil	6 parts
Perfume	.9 parts
Benzoic acid	.1 parts
Bromo acid	2.5 parts
Colour	10 parts

Procedure: Proceed as before.

III

White wax	7 oz.
Spermaceti	1 oz.
Liquid paraffin	1½ oz.
Carmine	2 dr.
Perfume	q.s.

Procedure: - Melt the waxes over a water bath and the finely powdered carmine is ground in. Then mix the liquid paraffin. Now strain the hot liquid through linen and set aside. When the temperature has come down to 110°F, pour it into moulds to set.

Perfume generally used is about one-half per cent coumarin or any other suitable perfume material.

IV

Vaseline	15 oz.
Beeswax	10 oz.
Spermaceti	400 gr.
Carmine	6 dr.
Perfume to suit	

Procedure: Melt and stir. Allow to cool a little before adding perfume. Pour into moulds.

V

Paraffin wax	2 oz.
White vaseline	3 oz.
White beeswax	1 oz.
Ceresine	3 oz.
Titanium dioxide	1 oz.
Carmine	6 dr.

Procedure: Proceed as before.

POMADES

The pomades are much in favour as toilet articles. The chief ingredient in all pomades is a soft white basis of white wax, spermaceti, lard, suet, vaseline, etc. When lard, suet, vaseline, etc. are used they should be previously refined and made free of all impurities and obnoxious matters. Other fats such as olive oil, almond oil, etc. may also be employed in conjunction with the above to serve as the basis.

The Mode of Preparation

To prepare the pomade the first step is to melt the pomade stock on a water bath and then add the olive and almond oils.

Now the pan is removed from fire and when it begins to thicken stir in various scents in proportions at discretion.

In preparing pomades the manufacturers may note that an addition of soap improves pomades. Before perfuming add about 250 parts of soap dissolved in hot water and about 1¾ parts of borax to 12,500 parts of pomade stock. This renders the pomade as white as snow and very emollient, which is very difficult to attain by an addition of stearine. This pomade will bear an admixture of one-third water.

In colouring pomades use is generally made of alkanet root, annatoo, gamboge root, chlorophyll, etc. It is usual to tie up the drug in a piece of coarse cloth and dip in a part of the pomade stock. Gentle heat may be applied and the whole squeezed from time to time. The strongly coloured stock may be diluted with ordinary stock to bring it to the desired shade.

I

Procedure: Prepared suet, olive oil, each 8 ounces, lard 4 ounces. Melt on a water bath, then remove the vessel, and, when it begins to thicken, stir in the following scents, in quantity at discretion: Oil of cloves, sixty drops; oil of neroli, twenty drops; oil lavender, sixty drops; oil of bergamot, ninety drops; essence musk, fifty drops; mix. A slight colour may be given to it, according to the fancy of the manufacturers with alkanet root or gamboge root.

II

Procedure: Melt 250 parts of freshly rendered lard and 25 parts of white wax at moderate heat and mix well with 200 parts of vaseline. Add 15 parts of bergamot oil, 3 parts of lavender oil, 2 parts of geranium oil and 2 parts of lemon oil, mixing well.

III

Procedure: Strained suet, ten pounds; white wax, three quarters of a pound. Melt, then stir well in bergamot oil, one ounce; lemon oil, half an ounce; oil of rosemary, quarter of an ounce; oil of lavender, quarter of an ounce; rose water, one pint.

IV

Procedure: Clarified lard, twelve pounds; clarified suet, two pounds; essence of bergamot, one ounce; essence of lemon, half an ounce; oil of lavender, quarter of an ounce; rose water, eight ounces. Melt the first two, then take the pan from the fire and stir in the essences.

V

Procedure: Digest 20 parts of coconut oil and 1 part of benzoin, in coarse powder, in a waterbath for 2 hours. Now have 1 part of carnauba wax, 1 part of ceresine and 5 parts of liquid paraffin melted over a waterbath. Strain the benzoated oil into the molten mass of paraffin. The product may be perfumed as desired with essential oils.

VI

Procedure: Melt 2½oz. of refined wax over a slow fire and then add 8 oz. of coconut oil. On cooling add 15 drops of oil of bergamot and 9 drops of oil of henna and stir well.

VII

Procedure: Take refined coconut oil 8 oz., white wax 2½ oz., oil of bergamot 15 minims, oil of henna 5 minims and proceed as above. Add alkanet root to colour.

VIII

Procedure: Take white wax 2 oz., refined coconut oil 12 oz., rose geranium oil 5 minims and proceed as above. Add tincture carmine to colour.

IX

Procedure: Take pure castor oil 8 oz., white wax 3 oz., otto of rose 5 minims, and proceed as above. Add tincture grass to colour.

Pomade A La Rose

Procedure: Lard, four pounds; suet, 1 pound; alkanet root q.s. Macerate with heat to give a faint colour, then allow it to cool and before it sets, stir in five ounces of rose water and add otto of rose to perfume.

Pomade A La Jàsmine

Procedure: Lard, suet, each one pound; oil of almonds, four ounces. Mix, then add spirit of jasmine, one ounce and a half.

VANISHING CREAM

Vanishing cream is so called because it disappears when rubbed into the skin. It consists of stearic acid partially saponified with alkali, the bulk of the fatty acid being emulsified by the soap thus formed. The main constituent is, of course, water and mucilage of tragacanth or agaragar to prevent the collapsing of the cream and the whole is preserved with a trace of an aldehyde.

I

Procedure: Melt 60 grams of stearic acid in a tared vessel of about 2 litres capacity, over a waterbath, and add 9 grams of sodium carbonate, dissolved in the minimum amount of hot water; to this add 7 grams of glycerine. Keep the mixture on the waterbath for one hour, stirring constantly, but not vigorously; add sufficient water to bring the preparation to 300 grams; then add 300 grams of the hamamelis water. Return the container to the water-bath for a minute or two, stirring the mixture until perfectly smooth. Pour into a warm mortar and beat to a foam. Let it stand for 12 hours, stir with a spatula and pack.

II

Procedure: Mix agar-agar 180 gr., distilled water 8 fl. oz., distilled solution of hamamelis B.P. 12 fl. oz. and allow to stand for a few days with occasional stirring until softened. Strain through muslin. Now heat together stearic acid 360 gr., oil of theobroma 360 gr., sodium carbonate 240 gr., distilled water 12 fl. oz., on a water-bath stirring constantly until combination is completed; transfer to a large jar and whip in the first solution with an egg whisk until a white foamy product results. Perfume to taste. Allow to stand for 14 days so that air bubbles may escape, mix gently and bottle. Large quantities may be made in an emulsifying machine.

The preparation will not show any grit and will keep long.

III

Procedure: Bring 1 lb. of glycerine and 1½ pint of water to a boil and add ½ oz. of carbonate of potash. Strain through a piece of cloth and heat the whole mass again. In the meanwhile have ¼ lb. of stearine melted over a water bath and pour this slowly over the first liquor. Continue heating till the mass is completely saponified. Then remove it and add 15 drops of oil of bitter almonds and 20 drops of oil of lavender. Beat the whole until cool and pack.

IV

Glycerine	$8\frac{1}{4}$	lbs.
Stearic acid (pure)	$4\frac{3}{4}$	lbs.
Distilled water	224	fl. oz.
Spirit	16	fl. oz.
Liquid ammonia (Sp. Gr. 0.888)	$4\frac{3}{4}$	oz.
Terpineol	2	oz.
Synthetic Jasmine otto	$\frac{1}{2}$	oz.
Synthetic Musk Crystals	10	gr.
Phenyl acetaldehyde	6	minims.

Procedure: Melt the stearic acid on a water bath at 75.8°C. Heat 2 lbs. of the glycerine with 192 oz. of the water to the same temperature, add ammonia, and pour into the melted stearic acid slowly, with constant stirring. Mix the rest of the glycerine and water and heat to 80°C, pour this into the first mixture with constant stirring, and continue the heat stirring for about 15 minutes. Remove from the fire and beat till cold. Mix perfumes with the spirit, and add slowly, with constant stirring to the cream.

Owing to the air and water present, these creams sometimes dry up. To avoid this add glycerine, grease, agar-agar and tragacanth.

V

	All in parts by weight
Stearic acid, triple pressed	200
Potassium hydroxide–sticks	14

Water	800
Carbitol	40
Perfume	10

Procedure: Dissolve the perfume in the carbitol and beat it into the cream at 20° Centigrade. To obtain a softer cream decrease the fatty acid and increase the potash.

VI

	All in parts by weight
Stearic acid	180
Potassium carbonate crystals	12
Glycerine	50
Water	750
Bergamot oil	2
Lavender oil	1
Ylang-ylang oil	1
Vetivert oil	1
Geranium oil	3

Procedure: Maintain the temperature at least 20 minutes, with vigorous stirring from the commencement of saponification. This will allow the greater part of the carbon dioxide to escape.

VII

	All in parts by weight
Stearic acid	180
Caustic soda–stick	9
Glycerine	50
Water	750
Coumarin	2
Sandalwood oil	2
Vetivert oil	1
Methyl ionone	6

Procedure: Dissolve the caustic soda in 360 parts of the hot water and add to the fatty acid. Mix the glycerine with the remainder of the water at the same temperature and stir in.

VIII

	All in parts by weight
Stearic acid	200
Fresh lard	20
Strong solution of ammonia .880	10
Distilled water	750
Linalol	5
Terpineol	8
Ylang-ylang oil	2
Coumarin	4
Oakmoss resin	1

Procedure: Add the ammonia to the hot water, stir, and pour the solution rapidly into the melted fats, triturating briskly all the time.

IX

	All in parts by weight
Stearic acid	130
Borax crystals	58
Sodium carbonate crystals	12
Water	740
Glycerine	50
Rose-geranium oil	9
Patchouli oil	1

Procedure: Pour the melted stearic acid into the boiling solution of glycerine, water, borax, and soda. Continue to boil until the mixture gelatinises. Cool and add the perfume.

X

	All in parts by weight
Stearic acid	180
Spermaceti	20
Triethanolamine	20
Carbitol	70
Perfume compound	10

Distilled water 700

Procedure: Melt the fats and heat the liquid to the same temperature. Mix and stir until cool—add the perfume.

XI

Witch-hazel Foams are made on the same lines as vanishing creams, excepting that a proportion of the water is replaced by distilled extract of witch-hazel, which is added to the already saponified fatty acid:

	All in parts by weight
Stearic acid	180
Potassium hydroxide	12
Water	260
Distilled solution of witch-hazel	500
Glycerine	50

Perfume with rose otto if desired.

XII

Peroxide Creams contain hydrogen peroxide at the time of manufacture, but it seems doubtful if this exists as such when they are used. The only means of securing the presence of available oxygen is by stabilising the peroxide with methyl parahydroxy benzoate.

	All in parts by weight
Stearic acid	120
Lanolin, anhydrous	20
Borax	30
Glycerine	100
Water	670
Hydrogen peroxide—20 volumes	50
Jasmine	6
Bois de rose oil	3
Styrax R.	1

Add the hydrogen peroxide while the cream is cooling.

COLD CREAM

Cold Cream is an emulsion in which the fat predominates, but the cooling effect produced when it is applied to the skin is due to the slow evaporation of the water contained. The base in general use is white beeswax, and traces of borax are occasionally added to aid emulsification. The perfume generally used is rose—either as aqua rosae or by the addition of otto. The method of manufacture is simple when borax is used, and consists of melting the wax on a waterbath, adding the oil, and warming the whole to about 80°C. The aqueous portion containing the borax is heated to this temperature and stirred in slowly. The perfume is added when cool, and the cream is potted liquid if a brilliant white surface is desired.

I

All in parts by weight

Almond oil	550
White wax	145
Borax	10
Water	290
Rose otto	5

II

Peach Kernel oil	600
Spermaceti	20
White wax	150
Borax	5
Triple rose water	215
Phenylethyl alcohol	5
Geranium oil–French	5

III

Almond oil	560
White wax	180
Lanolin, anhydrous	20
Borax	10
Zinc oxide—finely sifted	20

	All in parts of weight
Water	200
Rose rouge	5
Rose-geranium oil	5

IV

Mineral Cold Creams may be prepared with petroleum oil of 860 sp. gravity as follows:

	All in parts by weight
Paraffin liquid	570
White wax	160
Lanolin	50
Borax	8
Water	200
Geraniol	8
Phenylethyl alcohol	4

V

Procedure: Melt 60 parts of white wax and 100 parts of spermaceti over a water bath, then add 1,000 parts of almond oil leaving the whole on the water bath. Next add 10 parts of castor oil, then 300 parts of rose water, stirring continuously. Finally incorporate 2 parts of oil of rose, 2 parts of oil of geranium and 10 parts of oil of bergamot and place in jars. A trace of methyl violet may be added to ensure that the preparation retains its whiteness.

VI

Procedure: Melt 1 oz. of white wax and 1 oz. of spermaceti; add 8 fl. oz. of oil of sweet almonds in which 1 oz. of camphor has been dissolved with very gentle heat; then gradually add 5 fl. oz. of rose water in which 4 dr. of powdered borax has previously been dissolved, beating constantly with a wooden spatula until cold. Finally add 10 drops of oil of rose. This will yield camphorated cold cream.

VII

Procedure: Take petroleum oil 600 gr., white wax 60 gr., paraffin 140 dr., Eau de Cologne 30 gr., water 200 gr., rose water 200 gr., tincture of benzoin 10 gr., oil of rose geranium 10 drops. Mix the solid matter in the warm oils and pour into the mixture little by little, stirring at the same time Eau de Cologne and the perfumes. Stir well to get perfectly white.

VIII

Procedure: Mix together oil of almonds 425 parts, lanolin 185 parts, white wax 62 parts, spermaceti 62 parts. Make a solution of 4.5 parts of borax in 300 parts of rose water. Incorporate the solution to the solid ingredients.

IX

Procedure: Take spermaceti 4½ oz., white wax 3 oz.; fresh oil of almonds, 18 oz.; melt over water bath and pour in a slightly warmed marble mortar and stir briskly to prevent granulation. When the mixture becomes of the consistency of butter, triturate until it has a white, creamy appearance; add little by little, under constant stirring, a mixture of double water of rose, 1½ oz.; odourless glycerine, 1½ oz.; mix for 20 minutes, then add 15 drops of essence of roses and beat for about half an hour, when it will be ready for use.

X

Procedure: Melt 6 oz. of spermaceti and 4 oz. of white wax on a water bath. Add fresh oil of almonds 24 oz. and pour the whole into a slightly warmed mortar under constant and lively stirring to prevent granulation until the mass has a white, creamy appearance and is about the consistence of butter at ordinary temperature. Add little by little, under constant stirring, 2 oz. of rose water and 2 oz. of pure glycerine, mixed together, and finally add oil of bergamot 24 drops, rose oil 6 drops, oil of bitter almonds 8 drops and tincture of ambergris 5 drops. Continue the stirring for 15 or 20 minutes; then immediately put into containers.

FACE POWDERS

In manufacturing face powders the materials should be ground to a very fine state of sub-division and then passed through sieve of at least 100 mesh. For perfect results 120 mesh sieve is recommended.

After grinding and sifting, the ingredients are taken in specified proportion and a small quantity of such a mixture is put in a mortar and rubbed with suitable colour and then mixed with the whole lot and sifted twice to make sure that sub-division of the basic pigments has been accomplished.

Perfumes are next added by spraying the liquid perfumes on to the powder as it falls through the silk sifter. The amount of perfume used should be reduced to a minimum.

I

Procedure: Mix zinc white 5 parts; English precipitated calcium carbonate, 30 parts; best white steatite, 5 parts; wheat or rice starch, 10 parts; triple extract of white rose, 3 parts; triple extract of jasmine, 3 parts; triple extract of orange flower, 3 parts; triple extract of cassia 3 parts; tincture of musk, 8 parts. The whole is to be mixed thoroughly by repeated siftings. Orris root in powder may be substituted for the perfumes.

II

Procedure: Take pearl or bismuth white and French chalk, equal parts. Reduce them to fine powder and sift through cloth. Lastly add some artificial perfumes, as desired.

III

Procedure: A face powder of rosy hue may be prepared as follows: Starch 1,000 grams, carmine 20 grams, otto of rose 15 grams, otto of khus khus 15 grams, sandal oil 15 grams.

IV

Procedure: Take oxide of zinc 1 oz.; starch 8¼ oz.; essence of rose 5 to 10 drops; and carmine, as much as required for producing the desired tint.

V

Procedure: Mix 32 parts of bergamot oil, 10 parts of lemon oil and 6 parts of musk infusion with 500 parts of magnesium carbonate. Then triturate 5000 parts of rice starch, 3500 parts of calcium sulphate, 1000 parts of talc and 200 parts of powdered orris. Finally pass through a fine sieve.

VI

Rice Starch	600	grams
Maize Starch	200	grams
Talcum	100	grams
Zinc Stearate	50	grams
Zinc Oxide	50	grams

VII

Rice Starch	500	grams
Zinc Oxide	400	grams
French Chalk	100	grams
Magnesium Stearate	100	grams

TALCUM TOILET POWDER

Procedure: Talc, to be used as a toilet powder, should be in a state of very fine division. Antiseptics are sometimes added in small doses. As a perfume, rose oil may be employed, but, on account of its cost, rose geranium oil is probably more frequently used. A satisfactory proportion is ½dr. of the oil to 1 lb. of the powder. In order that the perfume may be thoroughly disseminated throughout the powder, the oil should be triturated first with a small portion of it; this should then be further triturated with a larger portion, and if the quantity operated on be large, the final mixing may be effected by sifting. Many odours besides that of rose would, of course, be suitable for a toilet powder. Ylang-ylang would doubtless prove very attractive, but its use is rather restricted on account of its high price

FACE LOTION

I

Procedure: Dissolve 10 gr. of alum and 1 gr. of zinc sulphate in a little water; mix 1 fl. dr. of glycerine with the bulk of water and pour in 1 fl. dr. of tincture of benzoin and 30 drops of essence of Eau de Cologne. Finally add distilled water to make 1 pint and mix well. The result should be a non-separable milky lotion.

II

Procedure: Mix 40 oz. of lactic acid and 80 oz. of pure glycerine in 5 gallons of distilled water. Now add 3 oz. of tincture of benzoin. Then colour with 40 grains of carmine and pour gradually a mixture of 1 oz. of commercial glycerine, $\frac{1}{2}$ oz. of ammonia solution in 3 oz. of distilled water. Heat the whole to drive off ammonia and mix intimately. Shake well and set aside for a day, filter and add 1 drachm of solution of ionone and a small quantity of kaolin. Finally filter until clear.

III

Lactic acid, syrupy	5 c.c.
Glycerine	100 c.c.
Tincture Benzoin	10 c.c.
Tincture of Styrax	10 c.c.
Patchouli R.	1 c.c.
Rose Synthetic	4 c.c.
Rose water to produce	1000 c.c.

Procedure: Dissolve the perfumes in the tinctures and add to the glycerine. Shake with 800 c.c. of water and then add the acid. Make up to volume with more rose water.

IV

Hydrogen Peroxide 10 Vols.	100 c.c.
Tincture Benzoin	10 c.c.
Muguet Synthetic	5 c.c.
Rose Water to produce	1000 c.c.

SUN BURN LOTION

Zinc Hydroxide (25 p.c.)	100 grams
Zinc Carbonate	70 grams
Corn Starch	30 grams
Glycerine	50 c.c.
Tincture of Benzoin	50 c.c.
Benzyl Cinnamate	2 grams
Heliotropin	5 grams
Tuberose Absolute	1 gram
Water to produce	1000 c.c.

Procedure: Dissolve the perfumes in the tincture of benzoin. Tint the powders with Armenian bole if desired.

HAIR CURLING LOTION

Procedure: Potash (Pure), 7 gms.; ammonia, $3\frac{1}{2}$ gms glycerine, 15 gms.; alcohol, 12 gms.; rose water, 550 gms. Wash hair with soap before application. Make the hair wavy in the wet; tie it up. The hair will curl on drying.

NAIL POLISHES

I

Celluloid film, cut small	250	parts
Amylacetate	250	parts
Acetone	750	parts
Eosine A		q.s.

Procedure: Mix the last two ingredients and add the first. Allow to stand until dissolved.

II

Stannic oxide	300	grams
Talc	300	grams
Osmo-Kaolin	100	grams
Tragacanth	2	grams
Glycerine	50	c.c.
Citral	1	c.c.
Water to make	1000	c.c.

Procedure: Rub the powders in a mortar with the glycerine, perfume and water, then pass through fine muslin.

FINGER-TIP COLOURING

Alkanet	$\frac{1}{2}$	oz.
Rectified Spirit	12	oz.
Rose Water	4	oz.

Procedure: Macerate for a week, add 10 drops of otto of rose, shake and filter.

A solution of eosine is also used; it should be made with perfumed spirits.

FRECKLE LOTION

I

Potassium chlorate	1.2	per cent
Borax	1	per cent

Potassium carbonate	3.7	per cent
Sugar	3.7	per cent
Glycerine	9	per cent
Rose water	20	per cent
Alcohol	10	per cent
Distilled water	51	per cent
Perfume	0.4	per cent

Procedure: Make separate solutions of the potassium carbonate and potassium chlorate and borax with small quantities of water. Dissolve the sugar in the remainder of the water. Add the glycerine and rose water; mix, then add the other solutions, individually, mixing before each addition. Add alcohol and perfumes.

II

Acetic acid	3	per cent
Lime Juice	10	per cent
Glycerine	6	per cent
Water	$70\frac{1}{2}$	per cent
Perfume	$\frac{1}{2}$	per cent
Alcohol	10	per cent

Procedure: Dissolve the concentrated lemon juice in the water and the acetic acid in the alcohol. Mix the perfume with the glycerine and add to the lemon juice solution, then add the acetic acid solution. Mix and filter.

ROUGE STICKS

Rouge sticks are very similar to lipsticks but these are slightly greasy and softer than the latter. The ideal lip rouge will rub on smoothly and also not come off easily. The carmine content should not exceed 20 per cent but the majority are made with much less. If a bright colour is desired, it can be obtained by the addition of zinc oxide.

General method of manufacture consists of melting and straining the fats and rubbing down the pigment in a warmed mortar with them, but for large-scale production, where a perfectly fine, smooth, and grainless article is desired, the warmed mass should be milled. Formulas are appended:

I

Liquid paraffin	300 c.c.
Lanolin anhydrous	150 grams
Ceresin (high m.p.)	350 grams
Carmine	200 grams
Linalyl cinnamate	1 c.c.

Procedure: Mix together.

II

Ceresine	300 grams
Almond oil	50 c.c.
Soft paraffin	500 grams
Zinc oxide	50 c.c.
Carmine	100 c.c.
Piperonal-vanillone	1 gram

HAIR FIXATIVE

Procedure: Dissolve 20 grams of boric acid in a litre of rose-water; add 50 grams of pulverised gum tragacanth. After several hours heat the mixture on a water-bath and filter through gauze. Perfume with 5 grams of oil of rose geranium and 2 grams of phenyl ethyl alcohol and finally add 100 grams of tincture of benzoin. Triturate in a mortar and pour into pots.

NON-GREASY HAIR CREAM

Gum tragacanth, pulverised	4 dr.
Water	1 quart
Alcohol, 90 per cent	2 oz.
Cologne water	2 oz.
Oil of cloves	12 drops

Procedure: Gently boil the tragacanth in water, strain through muslin, and when the mucilage is nearly cold, add alcohol, Cologne water and oil of cloves.

CANTHARIDES HAIR WASH

Acetum Cantharides	15 parts
Alcohol	150 parts
Rosemary Oil	15 parts

Bergamot Oil	10 parts
Lavender Oil	5 parts
Rose Oil	5 parts
Glycerine	50 parts
Water	700 parts

Procedure: Dissolve the oils in the spirit and the rest in water. Mix the two solutions and volume with water. Filter bright, using talc or Kieselguhr.

COCONUT OIL SHAMPOO

This is made by saponifying odourless oil with potash. Sometimes other fixed oils are added and these include palm, peanut, etc., but they have a tendency to decrease the foaming properties of the product and are only used in cheaper grade articles. Usually 1,000 parts of coconut oil require for complete saponification about 300 parts of potassium hydroxide. This is dissolved in 1 litre of water at about 75°C and added to the oil at the same temperature in a steam pan. Saponification can be tested by using phenolphthalein as indicator. If the liquid remains white, further additions of alkali are necessary whereas when it turns red more oil should be added. The heat is continued until saponification has taken place and the product is neutral. It is then diluted to 5 litres with distilled water in which some carbonate of potash has been dissolved.

Coconut Oil	1000 parts
Potassium hydroxide	300 parts
Distilled Water	1000 parts
Potassium Carbonate	30 parts
Distilled Water	2970 parts

It is now perfumed with any of the stable synthetics, such as linalol, terpineol, methyl acetophenone, etc., or such oils as lavender and rosemary.

LIME JUICE CREAM

I

Procedure: Dissolve by gentle heat white wax, $\frac{1}{2}$ oz.; oil of sweet almonds, 8 oz. Gradually add glycerine, 1 oz.; lime water (aqua calcis B.P.), 32 gr. with 1 oz. water; also add rectified spirit, 1½ oz.; essence of lemon, 2 dr.; essential oil of almonds, 5 minims.

II

Procedure: Take white wax 1 part, oil of sweet almonds 20 parts, lime water 22 parts, glycerine 2 parts, oil of lemon part. The advantage of this preparation is that it does not become rancid; on the other hand, it exerts a stimulating effect on the roots of the hair.

LIME JUICE GLYCERINE

I

Almond Oil	25	oz.
Glycerine	1½	oz.
Lemon Oil	1¼	oz.
Lime Water to make	80	fl. oz.

Procedure: Mix well by shaking.

II

Almond Oil	2	oz.
Glycerine	4	dr.
Tincture of Senegal	1	dr.
Lime Water	2	oz.
Rose Water	4	oz.
Oil of Bergamot	10	drops
Oil of Lemon	20	drops

Procedure: Shake well the oil of almond and tincture of senegal and then add the glycerine, lime water and rose water. Lastly perfume with essential oils. If the cream becomes rancid, add 4 grains of salicylic acid to each pint of the cream.

WRINKLE REMOVER

Procedure: Take white petrolatum, 7 av. oz.; paraffin wax, ½ av. oz.; lanolin, 2 av. oz.; water, 3 fl. oz.; oil of rose, 3 drops; vanillin, 2 gr.; alcohol, 1 fl. dr. Melt the paraffin, add the lanolin and petrolatum, and when these have melted pour the mixture into a warm mortar, and with constant stirring incorporate the water. When nearly cold add the oil and vanillin, dissolved in the alcohol. Preparations of this kind should be rubbed into the skin vigorously, as friction assists the absorbed fat in developing the muscles, and also imparts softness and fullness to the skin.

BINDI LIQUID

Carmine	5 parts
Gum arabic	8 parts
Water	10 parts

Procedure: Dissolve the gum in cold water and incorporate carmine.

BINDI STICK

Wax	$1\tfrac{1}{8}$ dr.
Almond oil	3 dr.
Carmine	6 gr.
Otto of rose	6 drops

Procedure: Melt the wax over a water bath, then incorporate the almond oil. Now dissolve the carmine in just enough solution of ammonia, put in a warm mortar, and add the bases. Next remove from the water bhath and add the otto. Lastly pour the mass in tin moulds.

LIQUID BRILLIANTINE

Castor oil	2 oz.
Alcohol (95 p.c.)	8 oz.
Oil of neroli	5 minims.
" of rose geranium	10 minims.
" of verbena	5 minims.
" of lemon	30 minims.

Procedure: Dissolve the castor oil in the alcohol and then add the essential oils one by one by shaking.

The liquid so obtained should be homogeneous.

CORN SALVE

Salicylic acid	6 dr.
Methyl salicylate	2 dr.
Wool fat	2 oz.
Yellow wax	2 oz.

Benzoated lard 11 oz.
Mix.

STICK COSMETIC

White wax	1½ lbs.
Tallow	3 "
Oil of bergamot	2 oz.
Oil of cassia	3 dr.
Oil of thyme	1½ "

Procedure: Mix the essential oils together and keep ready. Next melt the wax and tallow on a water bath. Now slowly stir in the essential oil mixture. Remove from the source of heat but continue stirring for a few minutes more until the mass is about to congeal. Now pour into suitable moulds.

II

Benzoated lard	1½ oz.
White wax	3 "
Oil of bergamot	1 dr.
Oil of cassia	10 minims.
Oil of thyme	5 minims.

Procedure: Melt wax, add the lard, and stir until creamy; then add the perfume and pour into suitable moulds.

SCENT CARDS

Procedure: Mix thoroughly coumarin, 10 gr.; vanillin, 10 gr.; heliotropin, 10 gr.; ionone, 10 minims; hyacinthine, 5 minims; essence of musk, 30 minims; otto of rose, 5 minims; rectified spirit, 1 fl. oz. Then soak a piece of blotting paper in the mixture. The cards to be scented are put in a closed box along with blotting paper for a day or so. The cards will imbibe the scent.

PERFUME TABLET

Perfume tablets consist of a compressed mixture of rice starch, magnesium carbonate and powdered orris root with combination of scents and essences, etc. The following are a few typical recipes:

Violet: Ionone, 50 parts; ylang-ylang, 50 parts; tincture musk, strongest, 200 parts; tincture benzoin, 200 parts.

Heliotrope: Heliotropin, 200 parts; vanillin, 50 parts; tincture of musk, 100 parts; tincture of benzoin, 200 parts.

Lilac: Oil of turpentine, 200 parts; lily of the valley essence, 200 parts; tincture of musk, 200 parts; tincture of benzoin, 200 parts. Mix.

SOLID PERFUME

I

Procedure: Melt 8 oz. of hard paraffin, and just as it begins to thicken add 1 oz. of kaolin with which 4 fl. dr. of concentrated essence has been intimately mixed. Finally pour into tin moulds of desired shape and size.

II

Procedure: Mix well finest plaster of Paris 4 oz. and powdered sodium chloride 10 gr. and make into a cream with water. Quickly add the essence, stir and pour into moulds.

APPENDIX

FIXATION OF PERFUMES

The following may be taken as illustrations of the number of the most suitable fixatives which may be used in conjunctions with sandalwood oil for a fairly wide range of perfume types.

Many of the substances here enumerated has not only fixative value, but contribute to the perfume.

Odour Type	Fixatives
Acacia	Balsams of Peru and tolu; myrrh; all types of musk, vanilla, cinnamic alcohol, hydroxy citronellol, civetone, indol.
Carnation	Amber, benzoin, benzyl isoeugenol, vanilla, musks, styrax, labdanum resin, sage oil, amyl salicylate.
Eau-de-Cologne	Ethylcinnamate, ethylanthranilate, Betanaphthol ethers, benzyl isoeugenol, sage oil, cinnamic esters, benzyl benzoate, musk.
Holiotrope	Benzoin, balsams of Peru and tolu, styrax, bromostyrolene, vanilla.
Hyacynth	Amber, styrax, benzoin, musk, cinnamic alcohol, indol.
Jasmine	Balsams of Peru and tolu, benzoin, styrax, hydroxy citronellol, benzyl salicylate, cinnamic alcohol, civet, indol, amylcinnamic aldehyde.
Lavender	Benzoin, styrax, musk, amber, clary sage oil, borneol, coumarin, phenylacetic acid.
Lily of the Valley	Aldehyde C_{11} orris, hydroxycitronellol, amber, terpineol, terpinyl acetate, musk ambrette.
Narcissus	Para-cresyl acetate, terpineol, cinnamic alcohol, amber, musk, benzoin, balsam of tolu, labdanum, musk ambrette.

Rose — Amber, musk, vetivert oil, patchouli oil, styrax, phenyl ethyl alcohol, cinnamic alcohol, hydroxycitronellol, ionone, benzyl cinnamate.

Violet — Orris, amber, ylang-ylang oil, vanillin, benzyl isoeugenol.

Ylang ylang — Benzoin, myrrh, balsams of Peru and tolu, para-cresyl methyl ether, benzyl alcohol, methyl isoeugenol.

A judicious addition of sandalwood oil is of advantage in practically every one of the above cases.

GLOSSARY

Agar Agar—China grass.

Alkanet Root—Raung pata.

Almond—Badam, vadam-kottai.

Alum—Phitari, phatkiri, sphatikari shib, zak.

Ambergriss—A fragrant substance found in the intestines of spermaceti whales.

Amla—Emblic myrobalan, amlaki, daula, gondhona, taupi, saljee.

Aniseed—Mauri, mahuri, sauriff, sewa, kuppi.

Bahera—Belleric myrobalan, bhaira, sagona, lupung, yella, tani, elupay, santi.

Bakul—Mimusops Elengi, mulsari, maulser, gholsari, borsali, magadam.

Bela—Arabian Jasmine, motia, mogra, malle, asphota, magra, nabamallika.

Benzoin—Luban, hussi, shambirani, kaminian.

Borax—Sohaga, tinkal, venkaram.

Caramel—Colouring matter from canesugar.

Cardamom—Elaich, ilachi.

Carraway—Ajowan, juvani, ajamo, owa, amam.

Cassia—Tejpat, sinkami, kikra, tamala, zarnab.

Castor—Arand, bherenda, eri, rendi, gaba.

Chameli—Catalonian Jasmine, jati, chamba, chambeli.

Champaka—Michelia Champaka, champa, shimbu, gandhaphali, chapha, shampang.

Chlorophyll—Green colouring matter from leaves of trees.

Cinnamon—Darchini, karruwa, kurrundu.

Cloves—Labang, raung.

Cochineal—A kind of insect known as kirmdana, kirmaz, kirandi, kirm.

Dolan Champaka—Magnolia Sphenocarpa, dulichampa, burramturi.

Fuller's Earth—Sajji mati.

Gandharaj—Gardenia or Cape Jasmine.

Ghanni—An indigenous oil mill.
Gul Henna—A kind of henna.
Gum Arabic—Gum of babul or kikar tree.
Henna—Lawsonia Alba, camphire, mehndi, shudi manghati, marithondi.
Indigo—Nila.
Istambal Kahi—An indigenous scent from rose water.
Jahuri Champaka—Magnolia Mutabilis.
Janti—Barleria, tadrelu, koileka, jhanti, jhinli.
Jasmine—Jasmine Auriculatum, jui, juin.
Kamini—Murraya Exotica, marchula, juti, kunti, naga golunga, makay.
Kantali Champaka—Artabortrys Odoratissimus, madmanti, manoranjitam, madan mast.
Keora—Pandanus, kea, ketuki, thalay, kaida, satthapu.
Ketaki—Keya, talum, ketaka, mugali.
Khus—Vetiver, bena, panni, valo, khus khus.
Kieselgurh—A mineral substance from a species of algae.
Lemon—Pati lebu, limu, limbu, nimbu.
Madhumalati—Echites Caryophyllata.
Mallika—Jasmine Arborescens, saptala, kussar, kusara, adavi malle, madhvi.
Marigold—Tagetes Erecta, genda, gendu, tangla, mentok, makhmal, guljafari, guljharo.
Mehndi—See Henna.
Musk—Mrighnavi, kasturi, mushk.
Musk Henna—Henna with scent of Musk.
Nageswar Champaka—Mesua Ferrea, nagkesar, nahor, nagchampa, thorlachampa, negchapha, mangal, naga sampigi.
Nitre—Sodium nitrate, sora.
Olibanum—Salhe, salai, kundur, luba, anduku, guggar, guggulu, dhup, chittu, bastaj.
Olive—Jalpai.
Orris Root—Irsa, sosun, bekh, ersa, irisa, bekh-i-banfsa.

Patchouli—Peholi, pachapat, panel, mali, pachhanadi, pokonilam.

Pumelo—Batabi lebu, bijora, papanus, sadaphal.

Quince—Cydonia Vulgaris, bilu.

Saffron—Jafran, kesar, kunkuma, kasmira-janma, saurab, kungumanu, kong.

Sandal—Chandan, gandha, sukat, santagu.

Sassafras—Cinnamonum gladuliferum, **Nepal** camphor wood, malligiri.

Sesamum—Til, gingelly, tir, tal, rasi, khasa.

Shephalica—Nyctanthes Arbor-tristis, har, siharu, seoli, singhar, gongo, pakura, kuri, khurasli, paghada, karchia.

Til—See Sesamum

Tuberose—Polianthes tuberose, rajanigandha, gulshabho, gulchari nela, sampenga.

WEIGHTS AND MEASURES

1 **maund (md.)** = 40 seers = $82\frac{2}{7}$ lbs.
1 **seer (sr.)** = 16 chhataks (ch.) = 2.057 lbs.
1 **pound (lb.)** = 16 ounces (oz.) = 7.7778 ch.
1 **ounce** = 8 drams (dr.) = 28.35 grams (gr.)
1 **tollah** = 16 annas (as.) = 180 grains (gr.)
20 **grains** (apothecary's) = 1 scruple.
60 **minims** (drops) = 1 dram (dr.).
1 **dram (dr.)** = 1/8 fluid ounce (fl. oz.).
1 **quart** = 2 pints = 40 fl. oz.
1 **bottle** = 24 fl. oz.; 1 gallon = 8 pints.

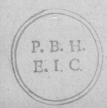